Your Health in the Information Age - how you and your doctor can use the internet to work together

Your Health in the Information Age - how you and your doctor can use the internet to work together

Peter Yellowlees MD

iUniverse, Inc.
New York Bloomington

Your Health in the Information Age -
how you and your doctor can use the internet to work together

Copyright © 2008 by Peter M Yellowlees MD

iUniverse books may be ordered through booksellers or by contacting:

iUniverse
1663 Liberty Drive
Bloomington, IN 47403
www.iuniverse.com
1-800-Authors (1-800-288-4677)

ISBN: 978-0-595-52775-5 (pbk)
ISBN: 978-0-595-51962-0 (cloth)
ISBN: 978-0-595-62828-5 (ebk)

Printed in the United States of America

iUniverse rev. date 10/30/08

Contents

The Author's Expertise

Peter Yellowlees MD is Director of the Health Informatics Program and Professor of Psychiatry at the University of California Davis. He undertakes clinical work at the University of California Davis Health System in Sacramento and is an internationally recognized expert in health information technology. He teaches both psychiatry and informatics to medical students, residents and graduate students from a number of disciplines, and runs an online graduate course in telemedicine through the University of California Davis Extension at www.extension.ucdavis.edu. He is in regular demand as an international conference speaker giving more than 100 presentations world-wide over the past five years. He has published more than 150 scientific articles and book chapters, including many on eHealth, has co-authored three books and received well over $7m in research grants. His full academic *Curriculum Vitae* is available at the web site for the Department of Psychiatry at the University of California Davis at www.ucdmc.ucdavis.edu/psychiatry.

Dr Yellowlees is Deputy Editor of the *Medscape Journal of Medicine*, and is on the editorial boards of the *Journal of Telemedicine and Telecare*, and *Telemedicine and eHealth*. He is a regular reviewer for many journals and has featured in several educational videos and films. He is involved in a series of exciting and leading-edge research programs involving telemedicine, virtual reality and data mining. He is a strong philosophical believer in patients having ubiquitous access to information any time anywhere.

Acknowledgements

I have written this book with the help of a great many people. Firstly I would like to thank the many anonymous patients and students who have taught, and enthused me about the many possibilities of the Internet in healthcare. The main reason I have continued to use the ever evolving health technology systems to link to patients when and where they need my help has been the positive response from them. I would never have even become interested in this area if my patients had not been so accepting of connecting with me over a variety of technologies since about 1992.

I have also received a great deal of support from my colleagues at both The University of California and The University of Queensland. These include Dr Robert Hales MD, Dr Don Hilty MD, and the many faculty and staff who work on the Informatics Graduate Program at UC Davis, and also Professor Peter Brooks and Greg Bain in Australia. I have had very helpful advice from Al Zuckerman, from Writers House in New York as well as from my past Brisbane agent, Margaret Kennedy. Rosemary Spencer taught me much about the process of non-academic writing, while Matthew Rickard assisted with excellent research and advice, always delivered with professional efficiency.

This book has been written with great support and love from my wife, Barb, who has always greatly encouraged me in this Endeavour. She is my greatest supporter and has enormously enriched my life. My ultimate aim has always been to make a difference in the world and to develop ways in which patients can more easily access good quality healthcare.

Preface

HOW TO USE THIS BOOK

Every day over 8 million adults in the USA search for health information on the Internet. Are you one of them?

Welcome to "Your Health In The Information Age – How You And Your Doctor Can Use The Internet To Work Together". This book has been written for the 140 million people in the USA who have already used the Internet to find health information for themselves or a loved one, and for the tens of millions of others whose medical records are now kept electronically by their doctor. This book is for all those who want to use the Internet to improve their health, who want to improve their relationship with their doctor, and who want to use the power of knowledge gained from their doctor and the Internet, to improve their health. It is written in a practical way to allow you to understand and select the right type of health information and use it in your relationship with your doctor in a way that is most helpful for you. I've tried to put a human face on the amazing technologies that are now available and show how we can benefit from them.

The goal of this book is to describe how you, as a patient, can best use the Internet to improve your own healthcare, and how you can do that by working with your usual doctor, and any of your other healthcare providers. Almost every patient that I see nowadays has already been on the Internet before my consultation with them. This is especially so if they have a chronic illness – and we know that more than 10% of the population at any one time have chronic illnesses like diabetes, heart failure, cancer, depression or substance abuse. Whether they have been on the Internet or not before I see them, I almost always recommend that patients look at specific websites to get more information about their health as part of their treatment plan.

But there is a gap in the available literature. I have tried to find a book that describes how to use the Internet, and other electronic communication technologies such as telemedicine and the telephone, to help patients work with their doctors. There really hasn't been such a book available, until now. That is why this book exists. I see it as a book that patients can use as a workbook explaining how they can get the best out of the Internet, and consequently improve their healthcare by working alongside their provider. It is a book that I hope you may have found because your doctor has recommended it to you, or perhaps you have heard about it from other patients. Either way, the book is meant to be used as a partner in your healthcare, to support you and your doctor as you make decisions, and implement your treatment for whatever health problem you, or someone in your family, has. This book can also be used as a resource for those seeking information about maintaining a healthy lifestyle and avoiding illness.

A WINNING TEAM

When was the last time you visited your doctor? What was it like? What happened? Who else was part of the consultation? Was your doctor using a computer during the consultation? And if so, for what purpose?

Think about these questions. Have you, like many others, seen your doctor in the presence of a third "person" – a computer linked to the Internet? Most doctors have rapidly computerized their practices over the past decade. They are very aware of the extraordinary amount of health information on the Internet, and most are fluent users of email, and many other software packages. Doctors have taken to the Internet like ducks to water, and use many aspects of the Internet for their own lives just like most other people in the USA. They use it to manage their practices, and many now also communicate regularly with patients on email. This is not surprising. Most doctors will use any useful innovation or new technology that presents itself to allow them to provide better care. They are very aware that this is the Information Age, and that they and their patients can greatly benefit from the amazing amount of healthcare information that is now at their finger tips, and from the astonishing access that they have to this information.

The fact that we are now living in the Information Age is recognized widely. It is national US health policy for all patients to have an Electronic Health Record within a few years time, so many doctors and hospitals are implementing such records to hold patient information. The same policies are being implemented in Britain and Australia. Large health systems like Kaiser Permanente are forming partnerships with commercial companies such as Microsoft to make health information more available to patients in the form of Personal Health Records – another way for patients to see, and contribute to, their own health information.

So what happened when you saw your doctor? How did he or she then involve this "third person" in the consultation? How did you feel about it, and did it help you? This is what this book is about. It is about how you, as a patient, can make the best use of this amazing new resource, the Internet, and the information available online, to work with your doctor, or any health care provider, to collaboratively become the winning team that is necessary to keep you healthy, happy, and fully productive in as many aspects of your life as possible.

YOUR RELATIONSHIP WITH YOUR DOCTOR – PATIENT EMPOWERMENT

There are a number of factors that are known to strengthen the therapeutic relationship that you have with your doctor, and they all fall under the broad heading of "patient empowerment". There is a truism in healthcare that "knowledge is power" and this is a key component of any good relationship – and this is something that can clearly be gained from the Internet. Another factor is choice. The capacity to make choices based on correct information, and on trust about the accuracy of that information, and where it is coming from, whether it is your doctor, or the Internet, or elsewhere. A third factor is responsibility – patients have to be aware of what is expected of them in the relationship, just as is the case for doctors – with any treatment program being designed to make the patient independent and able to take charge of their own lives and future treatment programs as possible. Finally patients need to know what are the expectations of any treatment program, who else might be involved (such as family, interpreters, other doctors), how can second opinions be arranged, and what are the possible complaints procedures if they are ever required.

All of these matters are related to knowledge and information, and all can be improved by working with your doctor and the Internet to better help yourself. 38% of patients in a recent study from the Pew Foundation reported being able to email their doctors in 2008, compared with only 6% of patients in 2003, but over 80% of patients said they would like this ability. We all know the importance of communication, and much of this book is focused on how best to communicate electronically with your doctor.

This is not a "hi-tech" book. It won't explain the intricacies of the Internet, or even how to log on. There are already many other books and manuals that do that and you should consult them as necessary.

Instead, this book will explain how the Internet can be applied to your problem or situation. This book is focused on what is helpful to patients. There are a number of books related to the Internet aimed at health professionals but they usually deal with specific technologies, mainly computers. This book is for the healthcare consumer-you!

In each chapter you will find case examples based on true situations which have been modified to protect identities. There are also checklists and self-assessments that you can use. Each chapter is designed to stand alone and deals with an entirely separate issue. The book is designed to be a practical information source about electronic healthcare, or eHealth, and acts as a guide to the best use of the Internet. It is not, however, a huge list of preferred websites, because these change all the time. Websites disappear, and reappear in a different format, and with ever changing content, continuously. What the book does do, though, is tell you how to search effectively for good quality information, and strongly encourages you to ask your doctor where they would advise you to go for the most relevant information for you. There are a number of other books available in almost all bookshops that act effectively as "address books" for health sites on the Internet, and I suggest that you look at them if you want to find large numbers of examples of topic related sites. A good example of such a book is "The Complete Home Medical Guide" published by the American College of Physicians, which has a comprehensive chapter listing useful Internet health sites.

As this book is written for you, you should treat it as you wish. Underline the sections that you find most useful. Write comments in the margins. Make your own notes as you read. Crease and fold the pages at important sections for easy reference. This book should not remain in pristine condition. It will probably end up being a reflection of you. Dip in and dip out of it! Read and re-read certain chapters or sections of special interest. Move from chapter to chapter. Think about the case examples and how they apply to you. Use the book as a work manual not as a conventional reading book. Try the exercises on rough paper, or gather some friends and family around and try them as a group to see how they relate to you. Give it to friends that you think might find it helpful, or to colleagues, or to your doctor. Don't just leave it on the shelf after the first read. Leave it lying around where you'll see it and pick it up again!

Finally, please do not hesitate to send feedback and your suggestions for improvements for future editions, to me at pmyellowlees@ucdavis.edu

1

The Web And Your Health - A Revolution In Health Care

I recently put the word "health" into the Google search engine. The search returned 1.32 billion web pages where the word "health" was mentioned. I do really mean the number 1,330,000,000 – more than a billion mentions. I followed up with other words. "Money" found 1.2 billion pages, "sex" 819 million, and "Microsoft" 868 million. What an amazing statement about the popularity of health on the net – more mentions than sex, money and Microsoft! And numbers of references now in the billions. When I did this same search in 2000, there were 27 million "health" references so this is more than a forty fold increase in the past 8 years. What an expansion of interest and use.

The business of eHealth on the Internet is expanding rapidly. Two recent reports from the Pew Foundation (www.pewinternet.org) and Harris Interactive (www.harrisinteractive.com) have confirmed that 75-80 per cent of United States Internet users utilize the Internet for health information and healthcare – that is around 140 million people. This is over 65% of the entire adult population of the USA – an average of 8 million people every day!. Not surprisingly those individuals with chronic illnesses, who have recently been diagnosed with a medical condition or who have broadband Internet connections use the Internet for healthcare more commonly than other Internet users, and their searches for health information is becoming a regular habit, often several times per month.

Business sees the healthcare sector as a particularly attractive industry that will benefit from web-based technologies because of its enormous size, inefficiency and information intensity. Moreover, the healthcare industry is particularly fragmented with a large number of participants, including general practitioners and primary care clinicians, specialists, institutions (public and private hospitals and diagnostic companies), health funds, pharmaceutical companies, retail pharmacies and, of course, patients.

John Chambers, from Cisco Systems, has been quoted many times as saying that "the Internet waits for no-one", and now that we have the rise of what is being called the second Internet revolution, with the influence of social networking and sites like facebook and youtube, the importance of the Internet has increased dramatically as it has entered the social fabric of our lives. We know that the radio took 30 years, and the TV 15 years, to build an audience of 60 million people around the world. The Web won 90 million people in its first three years and hasn't looked back so that there are now well over a billion Internet users around the world. If you want to get the latest numbers go to the Internet page on wikipedia.com, where continuous worldwide numbers of Internet users are constantly updated.

Countries like China, and regions like South America and the Indian subcontinent, with their large populations and economic bases, are becoming significant powers in the Internet world. I visited India in 2003 and while driving along the main road from Agra to Delhi was astonished to see broadband fiber being laid in hand dug trenches alongside the roadway, and to learn from my driver that this was now commonly seen as the whole of India was being rapidly wired. There are many different languages on the Internet, and while English is most certainly the most common language, every country has its own language based websites. It is a fascinating exercise to search for similar organizations or national interests around the world, and see how they are presented. I recently looked for all the organizations around the world interested in health informatics, as many are listed on the international medical informatics organization website (www.imia.org) and was fascinated to see how informatics was presented so differently in so many different countries, cultures and languages.

Many forces enable the practice of Internet healthcare - or as it is often called, eHealth – to advance rapidly, including the following:

- consumers are spending more of their own income on health, with an estimated increase in cost of 2.5% to 3.5% per year as the population ages.

- consumers are being encouraged to take more responsibility for their health, and to know more about treatments offered for them, their effectiveness and the track record of the individual provider or medical team offering the treatment.

- it is known that conventional health services are associated with many unintended injuries or complications, and government task forces in the United States, Europe and Australia have all strongly recommended more information technology involvement in the healthcare system to reduce errors and mistakes.

- health practitioners are now generally highly computer literate, and the medical students of today have grown up in a world where they have never known of life without the Internet. Many doctors have their own homepages, and the culture of health is changing whereby it is now well understood by both patients and doctors that patients can drive their care through accessing good quality information.

- the spread and increasing access to fast internet connections via broadband, which has led the whole internet to become so much more accessible than was the case when most people connected by dial up. Think how rapidly it is now possible to download video – films, TV shows, clips on www. youtube.com, family movies – and remember how long this used to take before the advent of broadband connections. I can certainly remember downloads a few years ago literally taking hours, whereas now most download times are measured in seconds, or minutes at the most.

- there were a series of highly publicized and funded Internet health portals developed before the "dot com bust" of 2001-2 that have survived and developed, with WebMD, Medscape and e-Medicine being probably the three most influential sites at a professional level. Major publishing companies have developed substantial healthcare Internet programs, and Google and Microsoft have recently entered the health industry with a bang, both focusing on building personal health records for patients, and working with premier health organizations, such as the Cleveland Clinic.

- the Internet itself is a major force, as it has literally become part of our daily lives. For example we now see kitchens routinely designed to include a computer area so that the cook can access the Internet while working there. Just look at the number of recipes and cooking websites available on the Internet. I wonder if you do what I sometimes do, which is to put a selection of the foods that I have available in the fridge into Google, and see what recipes come up using them. This is a great "decision support" tool for cooking, and is now starting to occur in the health area. A number of papers have been written where symptoms have been put into Google to see if the search engine can correctly identify the diagnosis – and it does so in about 50% of cases.

This book has been written to inform consumers of the advantages of the Internet in health, but also to allow people using the Internet, particularly when interacting directly with doctors, or other health care professionals, the ability to ask the right questions to ensure they are not being fooled. It will help people with the sorts of health problems illustrated throughout the book – those who have the problems illustrated in the following phone calls I have received:

A patient rings me. I pick up the phone with a feeling of dread. *"Please Doc, you've got to talk to my husband. I can't stand his drinking anymore. There's no way we can get in to see you. You're 300 miles away and anyway we can't leave the farm during lambing. I'm desperate. Last week he was drunk and I thought he was going to shoot us all. He keeps talking of suicide and how we're going to make ends meet."*

A call from another patient. *"I'm scared to leave the house. When I go out I feel like I'm going to have another heart attack. My chest pain just won't go away. I feel I have to always be near the phone to be able to call for help. I don't want to die. My kids think I'm daft and my husband's fed up. He's been great, doing the shopping and running the children around; but there's only so much he can take. I need some way of monitoring my heart that won't mean I have to call you all the time."*

THE INTERNET AND EMAIL

Today eHealth mainly involves the Internet and email, although videoconferencing (often called telemedicine) is also expanding rapidly, and is the technology that was mainly used to deliver online health in the past, and which I have used since 1992. In fact telemedicine is now being defined frequently as including videoconferencing, email, messaging and telephony – as all types of online technologies rapidly converge. The capabilities of the phone and video are being continuously merged on the Internet, with the use of Voice over Internet Protocol (VOIP) in audio or video environments through providers such as skype. Undoubtedly what used to be simply a telephone will emerge as a major health tool over the next few years, with the iPhone and Blackberry among leading products available everywhere. I certainly answer a high proportion of my emails with my blackberry, and access my schedule as well as make most of my telephone calls with the same device. Recently it also became the device that I attach to my laptop so that I can have continuous broadband access to my laptop wherever I am. We will eventually most likely move to a single digital platform for most distant health communications, but right now we still undertake our communications using relatively few approaches, as instant messaging and texting, while commonly used in daily life, especially by teenagers, have not had much impact in the health arena yet. This recent wave of interactive technology has already dramatically improved the ability of patients and their clinicians to communicate in more ways, and with more effectiveness, than could have been imagined even ten years ago. And the pace of change is escalating. It is estimated that the speed and power of computer technology is doubling every 18 months.

There are three main types of clinical interactions on the Internet; therapist/patient; therapist/therapist; and particularly patient/patient. Patients are using the Internet to help each other. Widespread access to the Internet and email has enabled great improvements in clinical and teaching services worldwide.

All clinicians at UC Davis have email so that patients can contact us easily if we wish that to happen, as I do. And patients do. And there are many websites where patients can access doctors who are prepared to prescribe and offer advice. I am deliberately not going to mention the names of any of these companies in this book because this is an evolving market, and they change constantly, but what you will discover is how to find and assess the sites for yourself. The largest of these web-based consulting companies in the USA supposedly has doctors available and registered in most states, and has over 4 million patients as subscribers.

The Internet is not a place for the unwary. Sir Robert Baden-Powell, when he dreamed up the Boy Scout motto "Be prepared" many years ago wasn't thinking of the Internet, but he might have been, because his warning is so appropriate. If you are looking for a doctor through the Internet, be wary, suspicious, hesitant. Thoroughly check out their websites to ensure they meet good professional standards and are not money making "fly by night" operations because there are still relatively few health professionals practicing fully online. It's always interesting to make regular checks on suspicious looking sites, say every two weeks or so. It is amazing how frequently they suddenly shut down or move – not the sign of a reputable operation. As long as you are careful, the Internet is a great place to find information and advice, although not yet a great place to connect with individual counselors or have an ongoing relationship with a doctor unless it is combined with a conventional face to face relationship. Talk with your doctor about how you may be able to communicate better with him or her via the Internet in preference to trying to find a primarily web-based doctor. And, as with any new adventure, go cautiously!

THE CHANGING FACE OF HEALTHCARE

A new millennium - a revolution in health care. Within ten years visiting most doctors over the Internet will be commonplace. Within the safety and convenience of our own homes we'll be able to speak to health professionals, access information on our health and receive support from groups of people with similar problems. Wireless videophones will be commonplace and we will be able to live in a virtual environment if we wish – able to contact our doctor, order groceries from the supermarket or set the security system in our home from wherever we are.

Most of the technical problems associated with going online have been overcome. What we have to do now is to change the way we interact and communicate as patients and doctors gradually get used to the capabilities provided by today's multi-media 24 by 7 environments.

As we spend more time online we must remember two core principles. The first is the complementarity principle - computers do well, what humans do badly, and vice versa. Computers never forget appointments or test results, while doctors are better at working out the meaning of an abnormal set of symptoms. The second principle is the importance of redesigning business processes before building new software environments – that one should not design new software to support an old inefficient business process. Many of our historical healthcare programs have assumed that a patient and a doctor have to physically meet to undertake a transaction, but of course that is no longer true in many instances.

We need to think differently, for example, about the doctor-patient consultation, which is what this book is about. At a basic level this consultation can be described as consisting of three information processes – data capture (the history and examination), data analysis (the diagnosis), and business planning (the creation of a treatment plan). Using the principles mentioned above we can now start to identify which components are best undertaken by the various humans involved, and which are best undertaken automatically or supported by technology. This is where the multi-media Internet has untapped resources and possibilities for patients and doctors.

Our population is ageing with "baby-boomers" demanding better quality healthcare. They are also determined to have home-based health care, and will pay to avoid going into nursing homes. At the same time governments are trying to reduce the escalating cost of health care by cutting back services as much as possible and closing down hospitals. Everyone recognizes that the use of electronic medical records is a way of improving the quality of care and making patient information more available where it counts, at the time of the doctor-patient consultation. We need to shift the center of gravity of care away from expensive hospitals and clinics, and back to the home.

It is not only cheaper to treat people at home and online, with less hospital bills at thousands of dollars per day, but patients can also become more involved in their own care. With a single keystroke patient, primary physician, specialist and home health nurse can be brought together. Many homes in the US have broadband Internet, or cable TV, both of which can be used to deliver electronic home care in future. Companies such as Intel are already developing technologies to be used in the home for the elderly in particular – for the baby boomers. These involve multiple health monitoring options – not only to collect obvious health data such as blood pressure, weight or pulse rates for patients with heart conditions, but to monitor patients with Alzheimer's as they move throughout their home, undertake survey responses from family members via television, and as alarm systems for any medical emergency. Telecommunications and cable television companies are the likely future infrastructure providers of tomorrow's health environment as they replace hospital beds with homecare accessibility. Care will be more available, better quality. Heath professionals more accountable and patients better informed.

THE NET IS WIDENING

Already 60-70% of American homes contain a computer, and according to the Pew Foundation, more than 80% of American adults use the Internet regularly. Most hospitals are moving towards introducing electronic medical record systems, and now have videoconferencing facilities that allows them to have high quality video conversations and interviews with experts or patients at other places, just as undertaken on news programs and seen on television every night. In countries like the Netherlands (88%), Norway (88%) and Sweden (77%) Internet access is higher than in the US (69%), which is currently only the 14th "most wired" country in the world, although the US is working hard to catch up. Billions of people around the world use the Internet regularly, many of them exclusively for email, although in Africa in particular the cell phone is the method of choice to access the Internet, and for online communication. The 69% of adults in the USA who have access to the Internet, has increased enormously compared with the figure of 23% in 1997. The Internet as a health care center, accessible to millions of people all around the world, is already with us. We now have younger generations, such as the current "millenials" generation, aged 18-25, who have never known life without the Internet, among the 1.2 billion users worldwide. This is approximately 17% of the worlds total population accessing a "place" that has only been in existence for about 15 years. What an incredible speed of take up.

The call from patients for more input into health matters continues to grow. The last decade has seen an enormous rise in the number and power of self-help and patient driven health interest groups, and they are all very aware of the need to have an online presence, and to communicate with their members via the Internet. These groups are using the Internet to provide information to their members and gather support for their causes through user groups, listservs, bulletin boards and online advertising.

At the same time computers are becoming more affordable. You can now buy a good quality home computer for less than $600 and the cost is falling nearly as fast as online technologies are improving. Several companies have developed $100 - $200 computers especially designed for the underdeveloped world in an effort to help developing nations rapidly catch up with the West, and to reduce what has been called the social digital divide.

E FOR EXPECTATIONS

The Web offers an amazing combination of immediacy, global reach, personalization and specialization. This means you can be the center of a world of information that is relevant to you, and which you have engineered. It has led to our expectations changing for basic service and product delivery. We now expect 24 hour global access, speed, do it yourself resources, personalization and customization, a large range of services and products, as well as the ability to pay online. In short, more choice and access, more empowerment. The convergence of technologies such as the phone, wireless, broadband Internet access, and digital TV is rapidly increasing the power and availability of information. The excitement caused by this convergence is reflected in the exponential growth of use of the Web, where uptake indicators are defying gravity.

If you want to discover details about the background, history and development of the Internet, look at wikipedia (www.wikipedia.org) , the multi-lingual web based free open source encyclopedia, which is a very widely used reference site, and which has essentially replaced the Encyclopedia Britannica, as the ultimate reference source. Wikipedia describes itself as follows:

"Wikipedia is written collaboratively *by* volunteers *from all around the world. Since its creation in 2001,* Wikipedia *has grown rapidly into one of the* largest *reference* Web sites *attracting at least* 684 million visitors *yearly by 2008. There are more than* 75,000 active contributors *working on more*

than 10,000,000 articles in more than 250 languages. *As of today, there are 2,378,273 articles in* English". *Accessed May 17th 2008*

Go there for almost any imaginable information you want. Here you can find that there were 93 users of the Internet from the Vatican City in 2007, and that this was 12% of the local population, compared with 210 million users in the USA, or 69% of the population in the same year. You can also read about Internet terminology, history, protocols, structure, common uses, social impact and access by region - all superbly well presented with links via the world wide web to multiple sources of information. Just remember that with wikipedia, while the great majority of information is carefully checked and is accurate, the core components of the encyclopedia are written by volunteers such as you and I, and we all make occasional mistakes. If you find mistakes on wikipedia, do please correct them.

For some time, Internet traffic has been doubling every hundred days, and the recent broadband shifts are increasing the speed of the Web by 50 to 100 times. Apart from the massive numbers of people predicted to connect to the Web worldwide, there are certain sections of the world where access is particularly common. Even Europe, which was relatively slow in the race to join the Internet era, now has widespread access and as we have moved away from not only having .com, .org and .net as the only domain names with the opening up of multiple other names such as .tv and .biz. The introduction of 24 hour streamed television, films and audio files on demand through a number of services such as iTunes, has led to us thinking quite differently of the mind-bending overall effect of the Web on global society. Many people, including myself, now use their computer like a TV or radio – we access podcasts (audio) and vodcasts (video) of the news and current affairs, download music and films, and watch sports from around the world on commercial streaming websites. We are certainly able to live and communicate in very different ways, and all from our home.

FEELING THE BYTE

In the USA in 2005 17,700 health care professionals provided care for 7.6 million patients in their homes, making over 80 million home visits that year. Most of these patients are elderly or chronically ill and by the year 2010 it's expected this number will have swelled even further. More dramatically, the home health care market in the USA, which was estimated to cost $34 billion in 1996, cost $53 billion in 2005.

But while home care is expensive, it's still less expensive than in-patient care where the average 2005 hospital admission lasting 5.8 days cost $28,000. The current annual cost of healthcare in the US is $2.3 trillion, or $7,600 per person per year. This is 16% of the gross domestic product (GDP), and these figures are predicted to rise to $4.2 trillion, and 20% of GDP by 2016. Inpatient accommodation alone in the US costs well over $1000 million a day; that's before any treatment costs are added. $3 for every American every day! Yet if just one person in every 200 could be treated outside an institution there would be an annual saving of $2 billion. Similarly another $1 billion could be saved by reducing the number of people in nursing homes by just 5%, one person in twenty. Obviously, it will be less expensive for patients to be properly cared for in their own homes using eHealth. We need to learn to spend less on health in the US generally as other western countries only spend about 10% of their gross domestic product compared with our 16% on health, and seem to have better health outcomes.

The move toward home-based eHealthcare will not, however, be driven solely by the need to cut costs. The rapidly aging generation of "baby boomers" will insist on more and better quality homecare and community services. As a member of the so-called "indulgent" and "demanding" generation, I have no intention of being hospitalized except under the most serious circumstances! When I am old I want to be cared for in my home, with my family around me, as much as possible, and I am very comfortable using technology to assist in that process.

IT'S *YOUR* HEALTH CHART

How often have you wanted to read what your health professionals have written about you? Through a shared electronic medical record you'll not only be able to read what your doctor has written. You'll also be able to check it is accurate and even contribute to it yourself!

For many years whenever I have had blood tests done by my doctor he has sent me the results at my request. However from 2005 onwards, when my healthcare providers implemented a full electronic medical record, I. have been able to log in to see the results online. It is so good being able to thoroughly check what is happening with my tests immediately after I have had them, and to track the results over time. Actually seeing my cholesterol results, and being able to link them with my weight and eating habits, makes a great difference, and has me much more involved in my own care.

The health homepage of the future will contain all your health records – it will be like your own health website. You will be able to make notes in it and collaborate with all types of health care professionals. Because it is on the Internet it will be accessible to you wherever you are in the world. It will be linked to health information, videomail, email and a range of related technologies that will allow you to see your own X-rays, pathology results, even your surgeons operating notes. Within a few years the following scenario will be commonplace:

"I've had a night of terrifying palpitations so, before going to work, I decide to seek reassurance from my doctor. I go to my home communications system and, via the individualized touch screen, press the videophone icon to speak to my doctor's receptionist, Mary.

Almost immediately she comes on screen via a secure high-speed video Internet connection. She compares my online diary with my doctor's and asks if I would prefer an appointment in person, either at the clinic or at my home...or by video, either to my home or via my laptop at work.

I decide to leave a note describing my symptoms in my shared electronic medical record for my doctor to look at when she comes in from her early morning home visits. She will either email or videomail me back if she thinks I should see her sooner than my scheduled consultation.

Keying in my password, I access my own record via the secure directories and write a short note about my symptoms. When I use the word "palpitation" it is highlighted as hypertext. I hit the hotlink and download a patient information sheet on "palpitation," developed by a university in England and recommended by my doctor. While I have my electronic medical record open I scan back and check what my doctor wrote the last time we met. I am pleased to see that her treatment plan is based on the clinical guidelines developed for my heart condition recommended by the physician I saw some months before.

Before going to work I take a few minutes to read the information on "palpitation" and remind myself of some simple techniques I can use to keep my heart rate steady during the day.

While this sounds futuristic everything in the scenario is technically possible today. The individual technologies only need to be integrated and used as part of an overall clinical process. This will happen in the next few years.

HOMECARE - THE WAY OF THE FUTURE

Online therapeutic techniques are about to radically change the face of homecare in the future. The following scenario is already happening in pilot programs around the world and uses equipment that costs only a few hundred dollars at each site.

"The tea smells wonderful, darling." Sylvia's voice from the bedroom continues, "Can you get me my medication – my pain is awful this morning – it's so hard to get my joints moving." Peter shuffles across the kitchen to the cupboard and takes out the medication dosette containing his wife's daily medication - each dose carefully worked out by Carol, their home nurse, on one of her regular visits.

He takes the morning pills for his wife's arthritis, pain and depression through to the bedroom. She's in so much pain...unable to move about much any more. He's thankful that he is still reasonably fit and can help her at home.

He'd been surprised at how easily she had taken to using the small video camera which now sat above the TV set. By using a broadband cable TV link they could see and talk to Carol and their doctor through the video camera and their own television.

Since Carol had brought the system they had seen a lot more of her. She used to come three times a week but was always in a hurry. It seemed she spent more time driving than visiting. Now she only visited the house twice a week but they usually had at least two other video sessions with her which Sylvia really seemed to look forward to. He couldn't understand why she dressed up and put on her make up for the TV sessions but it seemed to do her good!

It was also wonderful that their daughter, who lived too far away to visit regularly, had bought a similar set-up. Seeing her on the screen was so much better than speaking on the phone and, of course, it was lovely seeing the grand children!

Sylvia had always been a very independent person and refused to go to hospital. To monitor her pain and disability she agreed to fill in a weekly questionnaire of her symptoms in her shared medical records accessible on the Internet. This way Sylvia's doctor could monitor how she was feeling.

Once a week, during one of her visits, Carol arranged a weekly TV conference link with the doctor. This had greatly improved the communication between everyone.

This scenario shows how online health technology can both improve the quality of healthcare and save money. EHealth allows people to be treated in their homes and facilitates better communication between all those involved in the caring process. Studies have shown that home health nurses average five to six home visits per day when working exclusively from their cars in the traditional manner. If they used online health technologies they could probably make three home visits each day and six to eight video visits, so spending more time with their patients, instead of driving so much. Isn't that sensible?

POTENTIAL USERS OF EHEALTH

Almost anyone with a chronic illness, and many people with non-life threatening acute illnesses, can be helped by eHealth. Clearly people who are acutely and severely ill require urgent face to face assessment and interventions, such as hospitalization, may be necessary as a life saving measure.

Electronic consultations are happening across international borders, to remote rural regions in many countries, to prisons and nursing homes and to the physically or psychiatrically disabled within their own homes. Other beneficiaries of eHealth include people who are frequently on the move or on holiday. Some people simply prefer eHealth to conventional face to face approaches, or use it as an adjunct to their normal care, in particular to gain more information about their condition or to contact others involved in self-help or support groups. Consultations using broadband, usually satellite technologies, have been held to ships, in space and to airplanes as well as to rugged geographically isolated areas especially in America, Canada, Australia, China and other parts of Asia. And for those patients with an unusual or serious disease, who want to be involved in a clinical research trial, it is now possible to rapidly research the types of trials available, where they are being undertaken, and even sign up for them – all from home.

For deaf people the Internet is a special bonus. Unable to communicate by telephone as they cannot hear, the Internet enables them to communicate with their friends or their doctor over great distances. The same applies to the many people around the world who have aphasia, a condition usually caused by strokes, where people cannot speak because of damage in their brain but fully understand everything that is going on around them. Now they can communicate online, despite being physically unable to speak.

People involved in self-help or support groups who want to get to know other sufferers, or learn more about their illness are important users of the eHealthcare. The Internet offers an extraordinary choice of self-help, support and information options for patients and families from around the world. It is possible to find all manner of treatments, some bizarre, such as "urine therapy" where you supposedly benefit by drinking your own urine; "mainstream alternatives" such as homeopathy, acupuncture and meditation; and conventional approaches, especially huge amounts of information on medications.

And finally there are those who are involved in the prevention of disease, in research, administration and in community focused public health activities. In Malaysia planning is well under way for the Multi Media Super Corridor - a national health program using online techniques to focus on education and illness prevention. This is the way of the future. The National Health Service in Britain is undertaking what has been described as the largest information technology implementation project in the world as it makes electronic scheduling and electronic health records available to every person in the country at an escalating cost currently in the billions of dollars.

Many people now live in "wired communities," whole towns, such as Telluride in the USA, were given early online access as an experiment. Early evidence suggests that the online world can be extremely supportive for many, particularly for those who are lonely. It also seems that meeting people over the Internet may encourage more face to face interactions and a wider network of friends. With my unusual name I have already found several relatives on the Internet that I didn't know existed, and have been delighted to later meet them face to face!

But how do we relate to each other online?

RELATIONSHIPS ONLINE

Internet relationships have become common with a number of successful websites set up to create introductions. It is no longer unusual to speak to couples who say that they "met on the Internet". Online relationships have been explored in detail by Esther Gwinnell, MD, a psychiatrist from Oregon, in her fascinating book "Online Seductions – falling in love with strangers on the Internet." She demonstrated clearly that it is possible to develop effective and empathic relationships online but she also outlined the potential pitfalls of such romances. This book was written in 1998, but remains a classic, because of the accuracy of her observations and predictions.

"Falling in love over a machine? Many people find the idea humorous or even ludicrous. Yet it is happening, and psychotherapy patients are reporting this phenomenon to mental health professionals worldwide....It has become important to explore the ways in which people fall in love on the Internet, and to understand the similarities and the differences between them and relationships formed in person."

While there is an abundance of excellent and accurate information available online there is also some horrendously biased and inaccurate information and anyone who is considering becoming involved with an online partner, or developing an online relationship, must be wary. This is particularly the case because it can be hard to differentiate between good and bad information, as some of the most potentially damaging information is produced in a highly professional way on excellently created websites. So how does one differentiate between the good and the bad, especially if you are looking for an online counselor or therapist? The easiest way is to check whether the therapists or website writers have published their work in international and reputable journals. This is not difficult to do. To determine these people's credibility, and the credibility of their websites, ask yourself these questions:

Are the doctors, or other health professionals, actually the people they say they are?

What are their qualifications and do they practice in an ethical manner in accord with clearly laid down standards?

Are you sure they are not going to literally take your money and run – probably to another homepage to fool more people into parting with their money?

Health education and illness prevention strategies are still the strongest online modalities at present with accurate information about health problems recognized as being therapeutically beneficial to patients, significantly accelerating recovery. But you have to be able to assess the online doctor, and their website, in ways that are critical, yet reasonable. This book will give you straightforward guidelines on how to do this.

Will eHealthcare Change Therapeutic Relationships?

The major problem with online relationships is developing a realistic view of your doctor or counselor that is not clouded by the electronic wizardry. The clinician has the same problem but also has to break through similar barriers created by what I call our "e-persona." There is developing evidence to show that we tend to act and communicate rather differently when we are online, particularly via email, where no visual contact is made, but the same is also true in videoconferencing where therapeutic relationships also seem to be different, even although both patient and doctor can see each other. Charles Zaylor, MD, a psychiatrist at Kansas University Medical Centre and one of the most experienced telepsychiatrists in the USA, told me,

"I have become more direct with patients using telemedicine. I don't beat about the bush. It is somehow a more practical relationship that focuses very much on what people are doing in their lives, and how I can help them with good advice"

Similar experiences have also led me to work in a very different way with patients that I see in my normal practice, never mind online. My therapeutic goals and objectives are now more overt and specific. I'm more open and honest with patients about what I believe are their problems and the solutions and, in particular, I give them far more health information. Being an e-doctor for many years has helped me be a much better face to face doctor, and I am very grateful for that.

WHAT MAKES AN EFFECTIVE ONLINE DOCTOR?

E-doctors still need all their traditional talents especially empathy, warmth, flexibility, understanding and honesty. But they need more than that! They need to understand the issues brought about by their own, and their patients', online persona. This is an extra complicating feature of the relationship. I now teach media communication skills to the first year medical students at UC Davis who are intending to work in rural areas. They enjoy these sessions and soak up the advice as they realize how important this is, and how much of their future lives as doctors will involve using communication technology, not only to interact with patients, but to receive continuing medical education as part of their life long education path.

In the clinical situation E-doctors need better communication skills, not only in an individual setting, but also in groups. They must be able to project their personality in a similar manner to actors. Some people seem personable and friendly face to face, but projected onto a screen they portray as much presence as a dead fish. Whilst media training can help, and can allow them to be less self-conscious about projecting their personality an extra 20%, some of these people may probably be better off minimizing their online work.

Of course some people never discover what type of online persona they have. These people are terrified of technology, particularly computers, and develop panic attacks and a sudden desire for a long walk in the country at the very thought of an online interaction! Luckily these types are becoming less common, and our fortunate younger generations, brought up in a world of technology, are much less frightened.

TELEPHOBIAS AND TELE-ADDICTIONS

We all respond differently to new technologies. Feelings of helplessness or anger against computers or other technologies can lead to *techno* or *telephobias*. These have many causes, mostly social and cultural, mainly affect females, but occur in varying degrees in up to half the population. Mark Brosnan, in his book, "Technophobia" has gone as far as to suggest that such reactions are a "legitimate response to technology." It has been suggested that telephobia may be age-related. However, the large number of retired people who enjoy using computers does not support this. This is important as it is the elderly, through homecare, who will be one of the sectors of society to benefit most from eHealth.

Solutions to telephobias are examined in detail later, as is the rapidly emerging problem of tele-addictions. Most people in western societies will have read of cases of tele-addiction or know of people afflicted by it. As with any new experience there is always a group of people who simply go overboard in their enthusiasm. The online world provides an escape for many people but it can interrupt normal social activity, family relationships and psychological development. The latter is an especially important issue for adolescents who can develop computer "nerd" like lifestyles.

Internet activities are especially addictive, although I prefer to call the condition "problematic Internet use" rather than "Internet addiction" as I don't see this behavior as a full blown addiction. Others disagree and there is a group promoting the "illness" of "Internet addiction" to the American Psychiatric Association as a disorder to be included in the next version of the Associations diagnostic manual. Surfing the net is rather like gambling – one always expects to find the ultimate homepage in the next few minutes just like one hopes to hit the jackpot. When we do find a great website, possibly after hours of surfing frustration, our gambling instincts are reinforced and we carry on looking for the next "big win". Email users often have a tendency to check their mail several times a day "just in case" there is something urgent. Evidence is now emerging that email may interfere with work and home efficiency - and enjoyment of life - if it is not carefully managed.

Fortunately there are solutions to the tele-addictions. If you are worried that you, or someone you know, may have an Internet overuse syndrome or a telephobia, I have included brief self-assessment questionnaires which will indicate your risk of having, or developing, these syndromes. In time we will all learn to handle these types of difficulties as online technology and therapy become increasingly common. And that brings us back to the future.

THE FUTURE

What will happen to eHealth over the next ten, twenty or fifty years, and how will the relationships between patients and their therapists change as a consequence? No-one can be certain exactly how, but change they will.

In the late nineties, Warner Slack, MD, one of the gurus of the health technology world, predicted that all medical services would move out of hospitals to places of patient convenience and that hospitals as we know them today would disappear. He called their replacements, which would be within walking distance for many patients, "clinhavens." These facilities would be outpatient based and have sufficient information technologies and clinicians available to enable them to provide comprehensive care. He hasn't yet been shown to be correct but we are undoubtedly moving in that direction, although more slowly than he would have liked.

The growth of the Internet in the past decade has been extraordinary, as has the extent and capacity of the wired and wireless networks that carry online data. We no longer generally think of "dial up" connections to the Internet – instead we link via wired broadband technologies such as ethernet cable or DSL (digital subscriber lines), or via one of several wireless approaches. I now have a super fast computer at home attached to the Internet via my ethernet TV cable, which also includes my IP (Internet protocol) phone service either through telephones or the computer (via skype). My laptop, on the other hand, is used wirelessly all the time, via a local wireless network in my home, or through my Blackberry when I am traveling. My iPhone has Global Positioning System capacity, so that I can always find where I am on a Google map, as well as download music and breaking news instantaneously. We have massive bandwidth available all around the world through broadband fiber services such as Internet2 which allow multimedia (differing types of media transmission – audio, video), multipoint (video communications use multiple points) and multi-rate (differing transmission capacity) services to occur, in contrast to traditional telephone networks which take only audio from one point to another. Future networks will be up to a thousand times faster and more powerful than much of the present Internet and some of the bandwidth being used for research is already mind-boggling. We are all equals on the Internet.

This multimedia broadband environment will drive the changes to healthcare over the next ten years. More and more eHealthcare systems will be developed and embraced by patients and clinicians alike. Technologies will merge, and eHealth will become part of normal health practice so that many people will be treated with a combination of face to face, and "e" health approaches. While these changes are inevitable the main obstacle to their acceptance is still the cultural and attitudinal inertia within the health system, as clinicians struggle to change their work practices and therapeutic relationships. It is crucial that patients know what is possible so they can make informed choices, and any resistance to the widespread use of eHealthcare is broken down.

I believe that eHealth and the Internet will radically change the whole health system and lead to much better health for all of us. Care in all its guises will be more accessible and of a higher quality, while health professionals will be more accountable to better informed patients. Doctors will all have their own home pages where they will detail their experience, their continuing professional development, their license details and the results of their treatment. Surgeons will detail their infection rates, oncologists their cure rates, psychiatrists their patient rated outcome measures and most doctors, their patient satisfaction scores. This is starting to happen now. You can go to the Medical Board of California website and look up the track records of all

120,000 doctors registered in the State of California right now – including me. I suggest that you do this whenever you go to see a new doctor to make sure that they haven't been involved in some disciplinary action or been found guilty of a transgression that might affect their capacity to practice.

The parallel developments of the Internet and the increasingly technologically savvy population and consumer movement will create massive changes in healthcare. These changes will be accelerated by the changing social conditions and attitudes of our times. The "green" movement will undoubtedly have a large influence on healthcare as providers and consumers begin to realize that saving gas, by traveling less to receive or give healthcare, is an important green initiative, and that an increasingly digital health system is also likely to be a less wasteful system. Energy and waste conservation will certainly be made in other ways, but with gas currently at just over $4 per gallon in the US, almost doubled in the past 3 years, there is an urgent need to reduce the costs and resources associated with travel, and eHealth is a great way to do that. These will lead to a more accessible, reactive, fair and friendly health system which is increasingly individualized and focused on the needs of patients.

There will be improved communication between doctors and their patients with more emphasis on collaboration and long term therapeutic relationships facilitated by these new technologies. Face to face care and e-care will merge and simply make care more accessible for all and eventually global healthcare systems, crossing boundaries, continents and time-zones, will emerge. The roles and training of doctors and other health professionals will change as they work not only differently but more effectively. Doctors and patients will continue to work together, as they have for years, but their will be a "third person" in the consultation – the Internet.

Health education and disease prevention will finally become central to the provision of healthcare and health research will gather momentum with the increased availability and accessibility of information.

More people will be looked after in their homes at the expense of hospital and institutional care and patients and health professionals alike, will have an enriching and fascinating experience traveling the path of change together for the ultimate good of us all.

What an exciting future for patients and clinicians alike!
To summarize:

Many forces are making the practice of Internet healthcare advance rapidly. They include:

• more consumer spending on health

• more patients taking responsibility for their healthcare

- the recognition that increased use of information technology in healthcare should reduce errors and mistakes.

- the increasing computer literacy of most health practitioners and computerization of their practice environments.

- the emergence of the Internet as a part of our daily lives

- an increasing number of companies are showing an interest in the health

This will have many significant impacts:

- The Internet will become a major component of healthcare, and will change the doctor-patient relationship in a positive way

- Patients will increasingly have their health information collected in electronic records, and will communicate with their doctors electronically

- Many groups of patients will benefit, especially those with chronic illnesses, or who are geographically or socially isolated

- Some people will find these changes difficult to accept, and may use electronic health systems inappropriately

- Electronically mediated healthcare prevention and monitoring will receive more focus

2

Who Will Benefit?

It is fascinating to reflect on the changing cycle of health care over the past two centuries. Two hundred years ago if you wanted to see your doctor would probably have written to him describing your symptoms. Your doctor, who worked on his own, and who was never female, would have written back prescribing treatment which may or may not have included leeches or bowel washouts. Confidentiality was not an issue. Your health problems were often very public knowledge! Doctors didn't carry out physical examinations because not only were they often socially unacceptable, they struggled to interpret the results.

However, from the mid 1850's there was an increasing understanding of the importance of specific physical and psychological symptoms and the health care system has gradually changed. From a highly distributed open community-based process, people began to be institutionalized in hospitals, and the confidentiality of individual health records became increasingly important. In the last 50 years there has been a gradual move back towards community care with the realization that community based health promotion and prevention activities are more effective in the long run than expensive hospital care. This change is being accelerated by the online technologies which allow health information to be distributed widely and easily. And so we have just about gone full circle as we move back towards a distributed community based system. The difference is this time we have more education, more information and more privacy.

But what about the changes that have occurred broadly across our society in recent times? As a baby boomer I find it astonishing that most first year University students today wouldn't know who killed JR. In fact, who was JR?

For them Michael Jackson has always been white, the *SS Titanic* was never lost and AIDS has always existed. They were born the year the Walkman was invented, do not remember the Cold War, have never seen black and white television, and have not experienced life without the Internet.

This is the world we live in. It's changing more rapidly that at any previous time in history. The way we deliver health care is changing just as rapidly.

COVERING THE TERRITORY

"Circuit riding" is a normal part of many people's lives. Lawyers, salespeople, marketers, engineers and teachers regularly travel great distances to service rural centers. It's hard work and disruptive to family life. Constantly staying in motels with only the TV for company is not a good way to live. Most give it away after a few years, leaving younger colleagues to take up the challenge.

For years I was a psychiatrist "circuit rider" in central Australia. Circuit riders are people who visit distant regions on a regular basis to provide all kinds of services. In my case I regularly flew out from my home town of Broken Hill with the Royal Flying Doctor Service to hold clinics in towns hundreds of miles away. One of the places in the vast Australian outback I used to visit regularly was White Cliffs, 400 miles from the nearest state capital of Melbourne and two hundred miles from Broken Hill. White Cliffs is a small opal mining town built on chalk where the summer temperatures are routinely over 110 degrees and most people live underground in excavated modern day caves.

White Cliffs resembles a man-made moonscape, and the nurse who traveled with me to the clinics uncharitably referred to the town as a "free range psychiatric hospital" – a reference to the number of paranoid people she believed hid in their bolt holes. It was an unusual little town in more ways than one. Not only did its inhabitants live underground but a surprising number of them were named "Smith" or "Brown" and were most reluctant to give me any information on their backgrounds! Needless to say there was no police station in White Cliffs.

Over the years my understanding of the town and its people grew, but so did my frustration. My patients never seemed to be unwell on the day I visited - they always seemed to get sick between times! This meant that when I arrived they were either better, often following telephone consults, had left town to receive treatment elsewhere, or had become so unwell, through having received no treatment, that they'd gone into hiding and couldn't be found at all!!

If only I could have accessed the online technologies that are available now I could have "seen" patients between clinics and treated them in the early stages of their illnesses. Through the Internet I could have provided training and supervision to the town's health staff. My clinic visits would have been more productive as I could have spent more time with patients instead of running around town trying to find people who were untreated and unwell. In short, I was chasing my tail!

In future the most common users of eHealth will undoubtedly be those patients who integrate virtual care with their normal face to face care – they will see their doctors in the surgery and in cyberspace. This is what I do with my own patients at present. There are certain groups of patients who will find eHealth particularly helpful whether they integrate it into their usual face to face care, or not.

PEOPLE WHO ARE UNABLE TO ACCESS RELEVANT HEALTH EXPERTISE IN THEIR COMMUNITY, ESPECIALLY THE GEOGRAPHICALLY ISOLATED, OR THOSE WHO NEED CLINICAL TRIALS

The provision of health services to isolated populations, nationally and internationally, is the single most important therapeutic gain for these patients in the past century.

Most health professionals live in major cities - often where they were brought up and trained. Comparatively few people from rural regions study health programs at universities and most of those who do choose to stay on in the cities, rather than return to the country. This means that many communities have inadequate health expertise, federally defined as health shortage areas, while the centre of cities may have "too many" experts.

This is particularly important for those patients who need a "high tech" approach to their health, or who have an unusual or serious disorder, such as a number of cancers, where there is no "best treatment" available, and many patients are encouraged to take part in clinical research trials. These trials only take place at major academic medical centers, but finally they are becoming more accessible to patients who live distant from these places through the power of technology. Not only is it possible to find out what trials are available through which centers on the Internet, increasingly the trials themselves are being offered partly at a distance, with patients and researchers communicating online. Go to the amazing clinical trials site run by the National Institutes of Health – www.clinicaltrials.gov – and have a look. I just put in the search terms, "cancer and Sacramento", and found complete listings of 42 currently recruiting clinical trials for many different types of cancer - breast, prostate, lung, brain, colon – all potentially available and accessible to patients in need.

While people who are geographically isolated are the most obvious beneficiaries of the online therapies, isolation in all its forms is still a major cause of human distress. Human beings are inherently social creatures and rural dwellers suffer more from depression and alcohol abuse than their city counterparts. Generally, rural people's access to eHealth is more limited because the telecommunications infrastructure needed to support telemedicine or good Internet access is still not always available. Even now many parts of my own state of California still lack access to fast Internet infrastructure. Fortunately, this situation is changing, and within a few years fiberoptic cables, wireless systems and satellites will make online technologies widely available.

PEOPLE FROM DIFFERING CULTURAL AND LINGUISTIC BACKGROUNDS.

Many technologies are viewed and understood differently by individuals of different ethnic and cultural backgrounds. Such individuals have very different access to information technology depending not only on an individual's race or ethnicity, but also their income, their education level and their geographical location. African American and Hispanic/Latino individuals tend to report more affinity for information technology than Caucasians, but have lower access to this type of technology, and poorer skills to use it effectively. When poverty and low socioeconomic status are taken into account, only the Hispanic/Latino group in a major cultural study actually had significantly poorer access to technology than the other two groups, Caucasian and African American. The question then became, "Who lives in areas of concentrated poverty?" The answer is often ethnic minorities, and this appears to be true in both rural and urban areas.

A parallel issue of cultural differences in interest in technology and its trappings has been demonstrated in cultural differences in the capacity to form online relationships. Despite little research being done on this issue, one study has shown that Asians, especially Koreans, were more likely to form online relationships than Caucasians. The circumstances faced by many ethnic minorities in the United States seem to set the stage for differences in interest in, attitudes toward, and experience with technology that will certainly influence the process of delivering quality health services.

And here the Internet offers huge promise via automated translation services. One of my research projects involves undertaking medical interviews in Spanish with non-English speaking Latinos in the Californian Central Valley. We then use the medical center interpreters to translate the conversation and add continuous subheadings, and are testing whether English speaking doctors can do effective diagnostic assessments using these sub-headed videos. If this is possible it will open the way for patients all over the world to be assessed by doctors from other cultures so much more easily than at present. Doctors from America will be able to treat patients from Africa or South America. French doctors will be able to consult with Australian patients. People in China will be able to be examined by Italian physicians. And as technology advances, and automated translation and speech recognition technologies constantly improve, so will the power of the Internet as a health transmission service increase.

THOSE LIVING IN POVERTY, AND THE POORLY EDUCATED

Poverty is the most significant single barrier to receiving culturally appropriate health care, whether in person or by telecommunications. Poverty not only affects the technology experience, often causing limited or complete lack of easy access, or access only via outdated technologies, but it also potentially adversely affects the experience of use as well as capacity to change health care outcomes. Community poverty is very common in rural areas; 14.2% of the nation's rural population is classified as poor, compared to 12.5% of the general population nationally. Indeed, 81 non-metropolitan counties in the United States have poverty rates above 30%, and 12 have rates above 40%, with Tulare County in California noted as the most impoverished county in the nation. These rates of poverty are magnified among rural ethnic minority groups, which on average suffer double the rate of poverty of their counterpart white rural populations. Rural white populations report poverty in 11% of their members, compared with rural African Americans (33%), rural Native Americans (30%) and rural Hispanic/Latinos (27%). Rural areas are known to spend less per capita on health than their urban counterparts, and thus are less likely to support a community health practice and less likely to attract and retain doctors.

Another major confounder across many studies is education level, which tends to be related to poverty, as well as to socioeconomic status, and which may be related to decreased use of appropriate health services. An individual's educational background may also be correlated with previous exposure to technology, which could in term impact their comfort and openness to engage in eHealth care.

The 46 million uninsured are a reflection of poverty and lack of education, and are a blight on our national conscience. As a doctor, the experience of discharging patients "to the streets" because they are homeless is something I still find dreadful. The fact that these homeless people are given lists of shelters or temporary accommodation does not cover the fact that it is well understood that the night after discharge from hospital many will likely be sleeping under a bridge out in the open. It is clear that we need to address these issues of poverty and education as we deliver eHealth nationally and internationally.

PEOPLE WHO PREFER TO RECEIVE CARE, MONITORING AND SUPPORT AT HOME INSTEAD OF IN HOSPITALS OR OTHER INSTITUTIONS

In America the national annual expenditure on home care in 2005 was $53 billion. At the same time hospital costs are also escalating, and world wide attempts to reduce these costs are being made by discharging patients as early as possible. This is managed care, an intellectually dishonest term if ever there was one, and in the US this policy of early discharge for financial reasons has reached extraordinary levels where patients can virtually only stay in some hospitals if they are actively and continuously suicidal, or literally unable to walk. Fortunately the worst parts of managed care have now been discredited, and the process of "managing" to reduce costs, as a primary goal, seems much less common.

Clearly, cost is one of the drivers behind the move to increase home care. Equally importantly, aging baby-boomers are now starting to develop a personal interest in home care as the generation ages and they take a growing interest in taking responsibility for their own health care. In the light of these changes it is inevitable that patients will demand tele-home care services once they understand how effective they can be.

Perhaps the greatest benefit of e-care is that people can be treated, monitored, and kept in their own homes. Any visit to the exhibitors floor at major health technology conferences now reveals many companies making all sorts of technological devices and tools aimed at this market, and for those with a specific interest in these areas I would suggest a visit to the websites of the HIMSS (Health Information and Management Systems Society – www.himss. org) or the ATA (American Telemedicine Association – www.atmeda.org). Here you can find companies advertising every conceivable piece of hardware or software, all designed to support care and monitoring at a distance. There have now been a number of books written on homecare, and how technology can improve this process and link patients, mainly the elderly, with their families. Richard Wootton, PhD, an international pioneer of telemedicine, has reviewed the case notes of 1700 patients being nursed at home in the USA and the UK. He estimated that up to 45% of home nursing visits in the USA and about 15% of British could be made via telemedicine, and in future by broadband Internet. This suggests billions of dollars could be saved.

Equally importantly, those involved in current home health programs report almost universal patient satisfaction with the services. In *Cybermedicine* Warner Slack MD suggested:

"Gradually all medical services will move out of the hospital to places of convenience to the patient...Using interactive computing in their homes, patients themselves will manage medical problems...Doctors will make house calls. Clinicians and patients will know each others' names and will work together as friends."

So what are some of the applications of eHealth in the home? There are so many that I shall highlight just a few. The breakthrough program that first created clear scientific evidence of cost and clinical effectiveness of TeleHomecare was the Kaiser Permanente telemedicine nursing service run by Barb Johnston which was developed as a research pilot program..

This research program started in 1996 and incorporated over twenty home care monitors being used by a nursing team at any one time. The home care system was used mainly for patients with chronic physical illnesses – heart and lung disease, terminal cancer, severe diabetes – but people with chronic depression, anxiety and major social and psychological disorders were also treated. The program markedly reduced the "down" time that nurses spent in physically traveling between patients, increased their productivity from five to six visits a day to 15 to 20 video visits a day and also reduced the number of patients who were hospitalized. One of the most important findings of the program was how well accepted the idea of using technology to access health services was to homebound frail and elderly seniors. These people who were sick at home embraced the easy to use home video systems and were happy to be able to *connect* with the nurses so conveniently. The patients liked the fact that they could see and talk to their nurses over the videosystem and the nurse could check their vital signs remotely. In a review of quality of care in homehealth published in 2006 Barb Johnston wrote:

"The cost of this care typically is lower in the home than in other settings. Research has shown that home eHealthcare is an efficacious tool. Widespread adoption of information technology is now regarded as a path to improving healthcare and to achieving the Institute of Medicine's six quality aims for

redesigning care." She noted that these quality categories require health to be *"safe, timely, effective, efficient, equitable and patient centered".*

While there are many highly successful home health systems in the US, especially the ones managed by the Department of Veterans Affairs, which incorporate their electronic medical record, one of the longest running home technology systems is in Italy. This Italian telephone mediated home monitoring service has been functioning since 1987 and helps meet the medical, social and psychological needs of over 25,000 home-bound patients using a telephone call centre and home monitoring system. One of the fascinating outcomes of this service has been a much lower than expected suicide rate for that group of patients as they have gained so much support and confidence from knowing that their medical problems, mainly heart disease, are being carefully monitored.

PEOPLE ON SHIPS, AIRPLANES, SUBMARINES OR SPACECRAFT OR WHO ARE IN PLACES WHERE THEY CAN'T ACCESS CONVENTIONAL HEALTH CARE.

The world is already dotted with satellites that form a global communications network – look at the attempt by President Reagan to create a satellite based defense umbrella, and the amazing work of NASA on the Space Station. We can now look literally into our back yards using Google Earth, and see astonishing pictures of weather systems every day on the news. Who has not seen the amazing pictures of Hurricane Katrina as it wreaked devastation on New Orleans? Originally developed for the defense and media industries, this network is now increasingly being used for health purposes. The US armed services use the extraordinary power of satellite communications to deliver health care all around the world, from the battlefront, to major hospitals strategically placed in a number of countries. If you want to look at some of their advanced technologies go to the website for the Telemedicine and Advanced Technology Research Center (www.tatrc.org) and see some of the extraordinary work being undertaken by this group under the inspired leadership of pulmonary physician, Lieutenant Colonel Ron Poropatich, MD.

I have personally carried out a number of video consultations using the same equipment that news reporters, embedded in US army units, take with them into Iraq and Afghanistan. These consultations were in very rural parts of California, where there is no broadband access, and involved physician assistants being trained at UC Davis literally carrying all the satellite receiving equipment in suitcases as they moved around these isolated areas. It took them only about 15 minutes to set up the systems, wherever they wanted, and then they were able to connect via satellite to physicians like myself at the academic medical center in Sacramento. A number of commercial companies have been set up to deliver satellite technologies for Internet, video and audio, and more companies and organizations will undoubtedly enter this market soon. It is now possible to communicate with patients, and monitor their vital signs and psychological status on aircraft, oil rigs, ships and in the most remote parts of the world and send the information to relevant hospitals or, in particular, military health care institutions. The following are some of the examples of more extreme forms of eHealth that have occurred over the years:

a. North Sea oil rigs and platforms

A paramedic on an oil rig wearing a headset with miniature video camera, small TV screen and a two-way audio link examines a patient. The data was fed via satellite and land lines to the Accident and Emergency Department at the Aberdeen Royal Infirmary in Scotland where the relevant specialist advised on the patient's condition.

b. Sea Med

Sea Med was a program that started in 1998 and was originally run from the Cedars Sinai Medical Centre to provide health assistance to the many people are at sea. Sea Med estimated there are over 6,000 super or mega private yachts, none with any medical capability.Worldwide there are also over 100 cruise line companies carrying on average 400,000 passengers with an average age of 52 and variable medical support. Within the Merchant Marine Navy around the world there are a further 40,000 ships with over 300,000 crew members at sea every day. Minimal or non-existent medical care is provided for these people. Of course the large number of naval fleets at sea do often have very significant medical support on board. Overall well over 1 million people are at sea every day who could potentially be treated by eHealth. A number of companies have moved into this space transmitting via gyro stabilized satellite antennae mounted on ships, they can carry out medical consultations with people aboard ships through high quality video imagery, assisted with wireless satellite phones as necessary. Each ship is equipped with medical equipment and a drug inventory, very much like the Royal Flying Doctor Service has done into outback homes in Australia since 1927.

c. Climbers on Everest

Following the tragic deaths of 12 climbers on Mt Everest in March 1996, an expedition in 1998 successfully incorporated a trial of eHealth technologies. The climbers were equipped with monitoring and telecommunications devices which successfully transmitted back much useful health information. Several climbers also swallowed capsules which transmitted information on their core body temperature back through base camp to Yale-New Haven Hospital. Hopefully the knowledge gained about the effect of extreme climates on humans will prevent further deaths.

d. NASA and the Spacebridge to Russia

The National Aeronautics and Space Administration (NASA) and the Russian Space Agency started joint development of a medical education and consultation program in 1996 through the Spacebridge to Russia program. It was always intended that this would eventually develop into a program that would allow patients and clinicians at a number of centers in the USA and Russia to interact in real time audio and video over the Internet. And this is what has happened with a number of programs now linking the US and various countries that were part of the soviet block to provide health education and care. Take a trip yourself to www.nasa.gov and see the incredible pictures transmitted from space made available to anyone as part of the NASA public education program via the many vodcasts and excellent historical reviews on their site. NASA has been a highly influential group developing much of the technology that we now use in our daily lives, and on which we depend to deliver good health care via Internet technologies.

GROUPS WHICH NEED SPECIAL INTERPRETING SKILLS WHICH AREN'T AVAILABLE LOCALLY - LANGUAGE INTERPRETATION AND DEAF SIGNING.

Deafness is very common. In the USA 0.5% of the population, or well over 1 million people, are unable to use a telephone, even with a hearing aid. The introduction of care on the Internet opens up a whole new world of communication possibilities for these people. Support groups have flourished on the web, and several doctors in America and Australia now use "signing" via telemedicine to communicate with the deaf. These sorts of services are increasingly available via broadband Internet, and a Google search will rapidly give you access to a large number of technology assisted programs for the deaf. Of course the use of email, and Internet access, where sound is not necessary, has thankfully already opened up a whole new world of communication for the deaf community. Videoconferencing systems are now being used by some hospitals to help physicians to communicate with hearing impaired patients. Call centers who have trained interpreters are including staff who can use sign language via videoconferencing technologies to link to various clinics as needed.

PEOPLE WHO PREFER E-CARE TO FACE TO FACE HELP, OR WHO USE IT AS AN ADJUNCT TO THEIR NORMAL THERAPY

There is no doubt that some people prefer to answer computer based, rather than face to face, questions and that many of us answer a computer program more honestly than we do when asked the same questions by a doctor. This applies particularly to questions that we feel are embarrassing or personal. Other people simply prefer the convenience of being able to communicate with their doctor online, and like to be able to do this for much of their healthcare, while at the same time going to see their doctor in person when they feel the need. That is certainly what I try and do for my own healthcare. But what about those people with stigmatized disorders, victims of physical or sexual abuse, persons with HIV or impotence?

A classic example is child sexual abuse. I was recently seeing a 5 year old girl and her mother via videoconferencing. The child had been behaviorally disturbed for several months, but delighted in telling me, to the astonishment of her mother, how she preferred seeing me on TV rather than all the men with "big pee pee's" that she said she saw on TV at her new child care center, where it was rapidly obvious she was being exposed to pornography. Up until only about 15 years ago, child abuse was believed to be very rare…in fact when I was training as a doctor in the seventies it was not mentioned in the curriculum at all! Yet we now know that sexual abuse of children is tragically very common. Given that in the past most doctors were males while most victims were females, it isn't surprising that female victims didn't report abuse to their male doctors. If we had had other ways to collect data in those days apart from face to face interviews we would have probably have become aware of the extent of the problem much earlier. You will find a lot of individual and group support programs for victims of sexual abuse on the Internet – hardly surprising given the personal pain involved, and the still high level of stigmatization.

Impotence is another example. Relatively few males admit to this problem in an interview especially if the interviewers are young, attractive and female. Yet impotence clinics that advertise in the media and set up fairly anonymous services are overwhelmed by clients, especially since the advent of Viagra, which interestingly sells in huge quantities on the anonymous Internet via web pharmacies! We all have our pride and find it difficult to admit our concerns and fears to others face to face. And the same is true for services for patients with HIV – this is a difficult area medically because it changes so much, so patients with HIV typically spend a lot of time searching for the latest drug regimes, and for practitioners who are able to prescribe and monitor such complicated groups of medications.

Other people simply find relating to other humans a chore, preferring, the relatively emotionless environment of the computer. In earlier days these people might have become hermits, living out their lives in isolated caves, or entering monasteries or nunneries to avoid too much human contact. Becoming a shepherd or farming an isolated patch of country were other alternatives. Today such people tend to be labeled "avoidant", "schizoid" or "socially phobic". They often find it difficult living in our varied and busy society but, despite their difficulty communicating face to face, they still have strong emotional needs and are likely to benefit greatly from the increased accessibility to health professionals online.

In my experience, the other group of people who really enjoy talking to a "doc in a box" which is how I introduce myself to them when using video for consults, is children. Many actively prefer online consultations. Kids nowadays are brought up with technology, and have a different feel and approach to the online world – for them it is a natural extension of the face to face world, and not something strange or unusual. It is just part of their environment, and they continue relationships online and in the 'real" world very comfortably, and with no real difference between the two. Look at how easily the average adolescent can message their friends – often carrying on several conversations at once, while also talking to other people in the "first" world. Look at the popularity of "Second Life" a virtual reality multi-user environment (www.secondlife.com) with over 8 million members worldwide, including me, and on average 80,000 people logged on at any one time. If you meet "Nash Baldwin" in Second Life, do say hello – that is my avatar! Look at facebook (www.facebook.com) and myspace (www.myspace.com) where social networking has become a mainstream part of many people's lives, but also check out wikipedia and its descriptions of the hundreds of other social networking sites. The influence of your children is certainly going to drive eHealth forward as they will require and expect to consult with their doctors online, and doctors from the same generation will be very comfortable with this approach.

PEOPLE INVOLVED IN ONLINE SELF-HELP OR SUPPORT GROUPS WHO WANT TO GET TO KNOW OTHER SUFFERERS, OR WHO WISH TO LEARN MORE ABOUT THEIR ILLNESS.

Loneliness can be particularly distressing. It is possible to be lonely in a crowd or in the center of a bustling city. Loneliness is especially miserable when one is unwell, confused, uncertain or distressed. It is a medical fact that mortality rates are higher amongst socially isolated, or lonely, people and that this risk factor is independent of other well known risk factors such as smoking, drinking, social class and level of physical fitness. It isn't known why this is, but most humans do have an intense need for other humans, for relationships, for friends and these things are good for our health. So when we suffer from chronic illnesses such as asthma, heart disease, arthritis, cancer or depression we tend to try to find other sufferers to communicate with and learn from. This has been difficult in the past. The Internet, in particular, is dramatically changing all this...enabling sufferers to meet one another and gain support and help from those who understand their situation best, fellow sufferers. There are a remarkable number of online support groups and many of their websites will be accessible through the websites listed in this book – or just put as precise a diagnosis as possible, such as asthma, breast cancer or arthritis, and the word "support" into Google, and you will find large numbers of support options. Then follow the guidelines later in this book for assessing the quality of the websites and their content accuracy.

PHYSICALLY OR PSYCHIATRICALLY DISABLED PEOPLE WHO FIND IT DIFFICULT TO LEAVE THEIR HOMES

This is the classic case of "if the mountain won't come to Mohammed, then Mohammed has to go to the mountain". In the past people who were paraplegic, had severe disabling arthritis, or extreme agoraphobia often missed out on useful therapies because they couldn't get to a doctor. (How little we appreciate our legs until we are deprived of the ability to use them!)

The addition of e-care to homecare initiatives will make a substantial difference. Finally these people will be able to receive treatment instead of languishing, without the best care, out of sight, and unknown to, the health professionals who could help them. Disabled patients can benefit greatly when they can communicate with their doctor using email for those "visits" that can be done remotely. This does not mean to imply that any patient should avoid seeing their doctor when an in-person visit is what is required, but rather to consider using email if that is all that is necessary. An example might be a paralysed patient who requires a wheelchair van to transport them to the doctor's office just so they can ask if they can change a medication dose. If the problem can be managed via email that can save time and energy for the patient. If the doctor prefers to see the patient in the clinic then the patient can be transported. It's still a clinical decision but as more technology evolves more choices are emerging based on what the patient really needs.

INSTITUTIONALIZED POPULATIONS, SUCH AS PRISONERS, OR ELDERLY PEOPLE IN NURSING HOMES

EHealth systems, at present using telemedicine, increasingly using broadband on the net, are now regularly used in American prisons and are often linked to academic medical centers. Examples of prison online health systems are found in Texas, North Carolina, California and Ohio. Here eHealth is used for almost all types of health care, allowing nurses and other providers in the prisons to work with medical specialists to diagnose and treat prisoners. The Texas system is simply huge, with over 60,000 consultations, mainly for primary care, provided each year. Online healthcare allows prisoners much better access to high quality health professionals than would otherwise be possible and at a much reduced cost to the institutions. It would not be practical for individual prisons to recruit multiple specialists, such as orthopedists or infection disease physicians, but with telemedicine each prison clinic can link to specialist's clinics when they are needed. If a prisoners breaks his leg he can have the x-ray done in the prison clinic. The x-ray is viewed online by the orthopedist miles away and the real-time consultation can be done through telemedicine so that the specialist can see and talk with the prisoner and their nurse without anyone traveling. Without these services it would be hard to deliver the constitutional right of prisoners to quality healthcare.

Nursing homes are another area where e-care is being developed. In America and Australia a series of low end videoconferencing systems using ordinary phone lines (POTS – Plain Old Telephone System) were introduced into nursing homes some years ago to allow the occupants immediate access to their treating health staff at any time. Interestingly, many of the resident's children are also bought the equipment.which at the time cost only about $400 so they could keep in visual contact with their parents. Imagine how much pleasure this brought to elderly people and their families! These systems are rapidly becoming redundant, and are being replaced by Internet based systems which can routinely be used for video communications combined with information access, allowing e-care to be much more effectively delivered to many more institutions. In Japan the move has been to use cell phones for such care and communication, and there has been a huge focus on developing cell phones for monitoring symptoms, for video transmission, and for checking on the health of the elderly in particular.

PEOPLE WHO TRAVEL FREQUENTLY, VACATIONERS, OR THOSE WHO WANT TO KEEP IN CONTACT WITH THEIR DOCTOR AFTER THEY OR THE DOCTOR HAS MOVED AWAY.

A colleague of mine from England recently married his Australian fiancée in Brisbane. Unfortunately his parents weren't able to come out to the wedding from England as one of them had had a stroke. No problem. My colleague hooked up his laptop computer and included them in the wedding by videoconferencing to England! The wedding went well, his parents heard him take his vows and they were even able to videotape the entire ceremony back in England to keep as a lasting memory. Whilst they couldn't taste the wedding cake or kiss the bride they were able to share in the special occasion.

I have on several occasions agreed to follow up patients by telephone when they have moved to other states and are "between" therapists. Nowadays when I go overseas patients email me if they need to contact me while I am away. I still have contact with occasional patients I used to treat in Australia despite having left there in 2004 – by phone or email. They trust me, and often simply want to check that I am in accord with whatever treatment their current doctor is suggesting. In the past the only options for continuing care or advice were by phone or post, but today email is commonly used. After all why shouldn't you be able to access your usual doctor wherever you are in the world? And why shouldn't they be able to communicate easily with other clinicians you may need in an emergency? We expect TV news to bring us live interviews with people all over the world. We should expect the same level of service in the health domain.

PEOPLE INVOLVED IN PREVENTION, RESEARCH, ADMINISTRATIVE OR COMMUNITY PUBLIC HEALTH ACTIVITIES

The best way of improving our health is to prevent problems before they arise. Research shows 6 - 14 year olds are highly receptive to messages about healthy living. At this age patterns of unhealthy or health threatening behavior haven't become bad or lifelong habits. The Internet offers tremendous opportunities. Children love education delivered electronically, as long as the programs are interactive and stimulating and their teachers, supervisors or parents confident and knowledgeable. We have the opportunity to introduce lifelong protection, through early education of our children, against melanoma (skin cancer caused by excessive exposure to the sun), infectious diseases, particularly HIV and AIDS, obesity and various addictions. Online health prevention programs for children are currently being developed in many places around the world and will become increasingly available over the next few years. Visit the Office of Disease Prevention and Health Promotion at http://odphp. osophs.dhhs.gov/ for the most reliable and up to date prevention information from the US Department of Health, or go to www.healthfinder.gov where you can see, in my opinion, the largest library of validated health information on the Internet.

Researchers will also reap the benefits of eHealth. In the past valuable data was often consigned to waste paper baskets because everyone communicated verbally and made notes on paper. As shared electronic records are introduced valuable epidemiological data about health and illness patterns will be more easily available. Perhaps we will even be able to discover if mobile phones actually do cause an increased chance of users developing brain cancer if we are able to study enough people through these means – fortunately the evidence at this time points to them being safe.

IN THE LONG RUN WE ALL BENEFIT

In the long run we all stand to gain from eHealth even if we're not personally involved. This is because the development of e-care will lead to a general upgrading of health services. At present doctors tend to treat individual illnesses but online care will lead to increased emphasis on continuity of care, health promotion and illness prevention. There will be an attitude change in both patients and clinicians. These important issues will be discussed later.

Malaysia, with its policy of Vision 2020, has set itself the goal of "becoming a fully-developed, mature and knowledge rich society by the Year 2020." To do this it has developed the Multi-media Super Corridor, now known as MSC Malaysia (www.mscmalaysia.my/home). This is an area of about 750 square kilometers south of Kuala Lumpur, which is embedded with an extraordinarily high bandwidth digital communications infrastructure to link to centers of information, manufacturing and service provision across the country. The Malaysian government is encouraging what they call "technopreneurs" to integrate technological infrastructure and social systems and is using electronic healthcare as one of the "flagship applications". This initiative aims to keep people in a state of "wellness" through integrating seamless health information and cyberspace help services. The clinical programs will be supported by a series of educational programs for doctors and other Malaysian healthcare professionals. Hence the aim is not just distant medical consultations, but to develop genuine primary prevention programs across all areas of health which will include, for the entire population, individual "lifetime health plans." It will be a major social change! Singapore has gone one better, with plans to have every home in the country linked to the Internet!

At the other end of the scale, Nepal, a very poor country of 22 million people, immense mountains, isolated communities and very few doctors, is also starting to use the Internet to provide professional health education to its very isolated practitioners, to support them, and to keep them up to date with the latest medical advances.

WHO SHOULDN'T USE eHEALTH?

This is difficult to answer as there are no absolute contraindications to the use of eHealth and every clinical situation should be assessed individually.

You may have concerns about the online doctors' professional competence, ethics or qualifications. If your "therapist" believes that a 1 year course in navel gazing from the College of Emotional Harmony in Never Never Land is sufficient to practice psychotherapy over the Internet then I suggest you tell them to go straight back to Never Never Land! Always remember that Internet and email therapies may be offered by almost anyone. The message is "buyer beware" – check out the therapist! Follow the advice in this book.

If you are uncomfortable with the online approach and reasonable alternatives are available, then use them. If there aren't any alternatives then it may be that telephobia is the problem and ways of overcoming this are discussed later. Using the equipment shouldn't be a problem. With appropriate support and encouragement anyone should be able to handle it. Obviously if you can't get access to the necessary technology eHealth is not an option!

Your problems may be too serious to be treated online. This mainly concerns the possibility of acute medical, surgical or psychiatric emergencies. Whilst patients with these problems are often assessed online, face to face assessment, treatment and often hospitalization may well be urgently required.

In a crisis you should be able to easily obtain help locally if your online doctor is not contactable. Ideally, of course, your online and face to face doctor should be the same person, with you making the choice as to whether you "see" them face to face or via the Internet. Competent doctors will always make certain that emergency back up is available locally if they are away or unavailable. Occasionally this may not be possible if you live in an extremely remote area.

WOULD eHEALTH SUIT YOU?

The following eight point questionnaire, taken from the key points in this chapter, will help you decide if you, or members of your family, or friends would benefit from some form of eHealthcare. Remember-eCare does not replace your regular physician's care and advice. You should discuss your health needs with your own doctor including information and services that may be available online.

Try it out.

- Do you have access to the Internet

- Will you feel comfortable communicating electronically?

- Are you geographically isolated from the health services you need?

- In the event of your not being able to contact your online doctor in a crisis, do you have access to a doctor in your local community?

- Do you have a physical or psychiatric disorder that makes it difficult for you to leave your home or community to receive treatment?

- Would you prefer to be treated at home, at work or school, or in your local community rather than having to travel for care?

- Would you like to communicate with people with the same health needs as you?

- Would you like more information about your health?

The more positive answers you have given, the more likely you are to benefit from eHealth. Remember, there are no absolute contraindications apart from not having the right equipment to access the Internet! And of course the best approach is to combine your Internet care with in-person visits and the expertise of your usual face to face doctor.

3

Online Hardware And Software

CYCLES OF DISCOVERY

All innovations in health tend to go through a typical cycle. When a breakthrough is announced everyone is ecstatic and the new discovery is hailed as the cure-all to end all cure-alls. But inevitably there follows a period of disillusionment - there are problems, the common cold hasn't been cured, early enthusiasts now wouldn't use the new wonder drug on their dog! But in time the innovation reaches the third and final stage and finds its niche market.

The Internet is a classic example. The Internet went through a period of uncritical acceptance in the nineties, having originally been developed as a communication tool for university academics, but while it is now generally an accepted, and for many people, an essential part of their everyday life, there is more concern about its potential downside. We are now using the Internet more critically since the advent of global viruses, the first major one of which was the "love bug" of May 2000 which wiped out hundreds of thousands of hard drives worldwide creating a damage bill of many billions of dollars. Internet security is a huge industry, with ex-hackers frequently employed to test new systems, and governments literally spending millions of dollars worldwide to protect their electronic assets. Who would think nowadays of not setting up a security package on a home computer – almost all computers come complete with just such a security package, with automated online updates and monitoring. Major companies, national governments and large institutions like Universities are frequent targets for hackers, often fully professionally trained and working overseas. At UC Davis, where I work, we have literally about 2000 attempts per hour to break into our computer network, mainly from automated attacks on numbered computer ports. These ports to the Internet are strongly protected, and we minimize the number that we use, as do most companies nowadays, so that very few of the attacks are successful, but the number is still mind-boggling. Even now though, most people who start using email still use it massively and uncritically before working out what it is useful for and what merely wastes time. The telephone is the same. Take teenagers - particularly females. The onset of adolescence seems inevitably to be accompanied by a passionate urge to spend most of their lives on the phone, whether talking or messaging. Luckily in time this phase passes and the phone is subjected to more rational use, especially when the bills start coming in.

Over the next few years videoconferencing will increasingly be provided through the Internet and email will be supplemented by videomail. We already can use Voice of Internet Protocol (VOIP) for global telephony or videoconferencing via most major telecommunications companies or specialist smaller providers like Vonage or Skype. This will make interactive eHealthcare far more available, and to more patients. But enough of the future, let's look quickly at the past, and the development of the Internet.

THE TECHNOLOGY

If you want to know anything about the Internet, how it works, what it is, the latest developments, glossary of terms, major players, listings of relevant books and links to an unbelievable number of other sites, simply go to wikipedia or for specialist information on technologies to www.whatis.com. If you haven't got ready access to the Internet I strongly suggest you go to an Internet café or library to look this one up. The visual explanations, in particular, are fantastic and it'll save you hours of hard slog trying to understand the Internet. If you put the term "Internet" into Google, as I have just done, watch out – there are 2.5 billion references - I strongly suggest you don't try and read them all.

In brief, the "net" is owned by you as a public collaboration. It grew from a small research defense network in the USA developed to function even if a large portion of it was destroyed by a nuclear war. When you link from your computer via a modem or cable to an ISP (Internet service provider), you connect to their server (essentially a large computer attached to the global telecommunications network). You use your browser (a small program on your computer – usually Microsoft Internet Explorer or Mozilla) to select the address (the URL – uniform resource locator) of the site you wish to visit. This is situated on another server anywhere in the world also attached to the public network - and away you go. This is "surfing."

The most widely used part of the Internet is the World Wide Web, (the "web") which allows you to link by hypertext, highlighted or colored text, to other sites around the world. This was invented by Sir Tim Berners-Lee, widely acclaimed as one of the inventors of the web. He was working as a physicist and wanted to be able to share data, and described his invention as quoted on wikipedia: *"I just had to take the hypertext idea and connect it to the* Transmission Control Protocol *and* domain name system *ideas and — ta-da! — the World Wide Web."* The most commonly used single application on the net is email, which for many people has virtually replaced letter writing, although many in the "millenials" generation prefer instant messaging (IM), and already see email as being old fashioned.

To access the net all you need is a computer, (or a phone, PDA, or one of multiple automated devices in the home, car or workplace), a broadband or dial up modem, wired or wireless connection, and an account with an ISP who will usually provide the software you require. It will cost you under $1000 including the cost of the computer to start up and a few hundred dollars per year to connect. This has to be one of the best value buys in the modern world.

CLINICAL USES OF THE INTERNET - INFORMATION AND LEARNING

The Internet is the largest and most disorganized library in the world, although the creation and development of wikipedia over the past five years, described by Dr Chris Shute MD, of the Mayo Clinic, as the "largest and most successful computing project in history" has led to an extraordinary highly organized online encyclopedia. Wikipedia has literally led to the demise of several major book based encyclopedias.

The Internet contains massive amounts of good information on every subject under the sun, especially health. However, it also contains huge quantities of misinformation, at best described as biased or warped. A few Christmases ago I decided to look for some historical information about "Santa Claus" for my daughters. Fortunately they were not looking over my shoulder because all I discovered were the remarkable sexual activities apparently enjoyed by modern day "Santas!"

There have been a number of recent studies looking at the way that Americans use the Internet for their healthcare, and how they go online to seek health information. The Pew Foundation supports the Pew Internet and American Life Project (www.pewinternet.org). At the website for this project there are a number of fascinating reports that are being constantly updated that are well worth reading. They are based on repeat telephone surveys of over 2000 American adults. Here Susannah Fox, Associate Director of the Project, is quoted as confirming that

"Information gathering has become a habit for many Americans, particularly those in the 55% of households with broadband connections. 78% of home broadband users look online for health information."

She continues; *"Medical professionals were the dominant source for people with urgent health questions"* and notes that *"75% of ePatients with a chronic condition say their last health search affected a decision about how to treat an illness."*

The other major source on American online health information searching is Harris Interactive, (www.harrisinteractive.com) which, following a survey of over 1000 Americans in 2006, has confirmed the Pew figures that about 140 million US adults have searched online for health information, which Pew noted was an average of about 8 million health people searching per day. The Harris survey found that most people (88%) thought that their searching had been successful, but also noted that only 25% of individuals thought that the health information they found online was "very reliable."

So what can we conclude from this data. Three factors seem to stand out:

1. Searching on the Internet for health information is a remarkably common activity in America

2. While many people find health information that seems helpful, most do not really know if it is reliable.

3. People trust doctors to deliver high quality health information

Now you know why I am writing this book. If you work with your doctor when you are using the Internet you are likely to find much better quality health information, particularly health information that relates to you, and your situation, and is not too generic. If you can also use the Internet to communicate with your doctor, then all the better, as that will further strengthen your relationship, and make it much more likely that you receive the best possible care.

Now lets move on to the subject of searching for quality health information.

QUALITY ON THE INTERNET

Before we can benefit from the Internet we have to solve the problems of information quality and information overload. The Pew Internet and American Life Project has highlighted this need in their 2006 report available from www.pewinternet.org, by noting that

"The typical search for health information online starts at a search engine (and) *includes multiple sites. Very few* (people) *check the source and date of the information they find."*

The good news is that many efforts are currently being made to create good quality sites that deliver "guaranteed" accurate health information. Examples include the National Library of Medicine (www.nlm.nih.gov) and the National Institutes for Health (www.nih.gov) in the United States, Intute (www.intute.ac.uk) and Connecting for Health (www.connectingforhealth.nhs.uk) in the United Kingdom and Healthinsite (www.healthinsite.gov.au) in Australia. A number of high quality private health sites are available, of which the most widely used are certainly those associated with the company, WebMD (www.webmd.com). The main WebMD site offers excellent information designed for professionals and the general public. The associated sites, at Medscape (www.medscape.com) where the most widely read peer reviewed online journal, The Medscape Journal of Medicine, is presented, and at eMedicine, a massive peer reviewed medical review collection of papers, also offer high quality information designed primarily for health professionals. The Medscape Journal of Medicine, (where I have a role as Deputy Editor) has according to its editor, Dr George Lundberg MD, over 8 million enrolled members around the world, including 1.5 million US MD's, many of whom read it regularly.

A more comprehensive Internet classification and coding system, as well as the development of better health specific search engines to "mine" information, are required as part of the long term solution to this major problem of finding good quality health information. Only then will doctors and patients be able to effectively obtain good quality decision support information within the time and process of a typical online or face to face consultation.

Despite this problem, and contributing to it, there are increasing numbers of health portals available on the Internet which focus on a particular topic such as epilepsy, a country such as Australia or India, a professional organization such as the American Medical Association or an entire business network such as America Online. The aim of these portals, unless they are being set up for mischievous reasons, is to ensure that the hypertext links from the portal connect to sites that provide only good quality information.

The key to finding good information on the Internet is still at this stage finding good portals. In this book I have quoted you the Internet addresses of sites I believe are of reasonable quality. Unfortunately, though, as sites are constantly changing, there's no guarantee that they will stay that way.

HOW COMMON IS HEALTH INFORMATION ON THE NET?

Whilst it is estimated that there are over 200,000 Websites primarily devoted to health, and that about 60% of people who use the Net have used it for health-related reasons, there is a simpler way of estimating how much information on health there is around the Web. And it's very simple, try for yourself. Just go to Google, and put in a simple and common term that relates to your area of interest. Then count the number of Web pages returned to you.

I did this for a series of common words and names in 2000 and show the results below, and then the results of the same searches performed in May 2008. As you can see I found literally millions of pages that reported using these words but the number of websites referencing them have increased exponentially in the last 8 years, a clear indication of the extraordinary growth of the Internet during that time.

NUMBERS OF WEB PAGES REPORTING COMMON WORDS
(numbers in millions of reported Web pages)

2000

Sex	10 million	Beatles	4 million
Money	9 million	Pamela Anderson	0.1 million
Microsoft	10 million	Bill Gates	0.3 million
God	4 million	Jesus	2.5 million
The Bible	3 million	Coca-Cola	0.3 million
Tax	4 million		

2008

Sex	819 million	Beatles	83 million
Money	1200 million	Pamela Anderson	24 million
Microsoft	868 million	Bill Gates	23 million
God	655 million	Jesus	248 million

The Bible	179 million	Coca-Cola	55 million
Tax	509 million	Britney Spears	92 million
		Paris Hilton	70 million

I deliberately chose these words because they are either in common use in the English language, or commonly reported to the issues on the Web. It is fascinating that Sex, Money and Microsoft all turned up around the same number of pages in 2000, yet by 2008, Money is clearly ahead. God, the Bible, Jesus and Tax all came in around at the same levels of interest and popularity, along with the Beatles, in 2000, but by 2008 God and Tax have surged ahead of the rest, and the Beatles, sadly, have slipped behind the relatively recent media phenomenon, Britney Spears. In 2000 rather to my surprise, Coca-Cola, perhaps a more specific search word than some of the others, and Bill Gates were much less popular than the other search words, but still were mentioned over 300,000 times, whilst Pamela Anderson, who has often been reported as being the single most effective sales person on the Web, via her sex marketing profile, only featured on about 100,000 pages. But all of these pale in comparison with Britney in 2008, and her publicity seeking colleague, Paris Hilton. And look at the increased interest in religion on the Internet during this time.

So what about health-related words? All I can say is, that they were amazingly common. Look at the table below. The term "health" which admittedly, can be used in a variety of ways, and doesn't necessarily relate purely to medicine, was shown on 27 million Websites in 2000, and on 1.33 billion sites in 2008! Much more common than Money, Sex and Microsoft. Mind you, for fun, I thought I'd have a look at the first Website that come up under the health search term and instantly found myself in a highly pornographic voyeuristic site! But that is the Web, and in particular, shows how careful you have to be, and how much overlap there is on general searches by topic. The other health-related words in the table are also extremely common but look at how their numbers have changed over the past 8 years.

HEALTH WORDS – Number of millions of Web pages found:

2000

Birth	6 million	Therapy	1.7 million
Death	5 million	Medication	0.3 million
Disease	3 million	Nurse	0.6 million
Hospital	3.5 million	Physician	1 million
Medicine	5 million	Therapist	0.2 million

Patient	2 million	Alcohol	1 million
Doctor	2 million		

2008

Birth	258 million	Therapy	190 million
Death	631 million	Medication	62 million
Disease	245 million	Nurse	118 million
Hospital	364 million	Physician	85 million
Medicine	365 million	Therapist	40 million
Patient	189 million	Alcohol	178 million
Doctor	322 million		

Compare these terms with the non-health items in the first table for 2000. Birth, Death and Medicine are all more commonly mentioned than God, the Bible and Tax. Doctor and Patient appear about as commonly as Jesus and Alcohol gets three times more mentions than Coca-Cola! By the time we come to 2008 it is obvious that there are two major changes. Firstly the numbers of mentions of health words have increased proportionately by over 100 times, which is similar to the non-health words in the first tables. Secondly death, taxes and sex are now all in the same range, with very common mentions of doctor, hospital and medicine.

Sure this is not high science. It is only a very simple example of the amount of potentially relevant health information on the Web, and how this is increasing at an extraordinary rate. But it's convincing.

LINKS WITH LIKE-MINDED INDIVIDUALS

The Internet allows people with similar interests, passions or problems to connect, interact and communicate, generally via email or instant messaging, after finding out about each other through conventional advertising in the press or via websites, bulletin boards, chat groups or Internet search engines.

One of my patients is a good example of this. Distressed by unusual symptoms of depersonalization…where she feels detached from her body… she has gained a great deal of support and information from the Internet. Surfing the net she discovered a specific research program on depersonalization in Europe and after completing assessment protocols for the project by email, was invited to take part in the research.

Contact with groups of fellow sufferers through the Internet has made her feel less alone and she has also learned of several unusual therapeutic options to reduce the distress caused by her symptoms. We don't know whether they will work yet, but the fact that they have been recommended by other sufferers has been most helpful to her.

INDIVIDUAL HEALTH SERVICES THROUGH AN INTERNET DOCTOR

This is cowboy country at present, although many companies and groups have been set up to try and provide clinical consultations on the Internet. Most of them have failed, and those that have not have usually either changed their business approach, or have taken to Internet prescribing. Relatively small numbers of patients are currently being formally treated on the "net" by qualified professionals despite the hype and self- promotion of other so-called professionals, although some companies do exist that seem to be making a reasonable business. They can be found via Google but they change all the time and I certainly couldn't recommend one at this time. However I'm certain that it won't be long before recognized treatments and consultations become widely available on the Internet. These will be a tremendous help to geographically isolated people who at present find it extremely difficult to access good quality advice and treatment. Advice on selecting a reputable Internet doctor will be given later in this book.

I had personal involvement for several years with one such company based in New Zealand, Doctor Global, which originally was set up to provide Internet consultations. In 2000, when the Doctor Global was very active, and before the dot com boom, I wrote the following:

"One of the companies being set up with a strong ethical and clinical base, is www.doctorglobal.com This site is an example of what is about to come. Of how common email consultations will be. Of how simple virtual consultations can be. And how a group of health professionals, mainly doctors, can combine to offer quality eHealth services in many countries and for a range of purposes. Doctor Global, set up by a New Zealand General Practitioner, Tom Mulholland, has eleven online clinics: General, Sexual, Heart, Travel, Nutrition, Allergy, Occupational Health, Mental Health, Asthma and Sports Medicine. I am involved in directing the mental health clinic and there are already considerable numbers of consultations being performed by the qualified medical staff who subcontract their services to Doctor Global, and who's photographs and professional credentials are shown on the site. Sites such as this which offer accountable quality ethically

sound health services are still uncommon – have a look at <u>www.doctorglobal.</u> <u>com</u> *as an example of the "best of the web."*

Sadly, Doctor Global was unable to sustain itself financially as the numbers of consultations undertaken were simply never sufficient to gain profitability and in 2002 it ceased undertaking consultations. The company then went through two further business transitions, in an attempt to be successful. Firstly it morphed into a "personal health record" company. Doctor Global had built an excellent software application to undertake online consultations, so it marketed this software environment as a personal health record. Unfortunately this did not work either, as the market for personal health records, as I write in 2008, is still in its infancy, and the company was ahead of its time on this topic in 2002. After some time spent on this approach, the company successfully moved into its third phase, that of selling a disease management software application, and has been involved in that field since 2004. It was fascinating to see this company start out as an attempt to be a clinical service company run by a group of doctors, and gradually become a software application development business with no doctors involved any more. This example is not unusual and the field of Internet consultations is littered with failed or changed business attempts.

Other present day health activities on the Internet include bulletin boards, discussion groups and mailing lists for health professionals and patients to communicate and exchange information. These are increasingly sophisticated and interactive, with more real-time chat events and webinars, and many incorporate video as well as the written word.

Continuing medical education (CME) will be a major growth area for professionals with more interactivity and voice/picture combinations becoming available over the Internet. The CME credits offered through WebMD, involving many video presentations, as well as online articles published by the Medscape Journal of Medicine, now make up for 17% of all CME activities claimed by US physicians. Most major medical centers and associations offer online CME. You can look at the UC Davis CME website (<u>www.ucdmc.ucdavis.edu/cme</u>) if you want, and there can watch many hours of fully accredited CME lectures, including more than a dozen presented by yours truly.

BUYING HEALTHCARE PRODUCTS

This is perhaps the most high profile, and most clinically problematic area. The sale of medications via the Internet is hugely profitable for those companies that are involved, but is a major ethical problem, and if it continues in a completely unregulated way, has the potential to cause much harm. Viagra is the drug that, classically, has sold well on the web. It is used to treat impotence, and many men who take it are afraid to discuss their problems with their doctor – it is much easier to get on the net and order the medication direct. The problem is that a drug like Viagra should only be taken after consultation with a doctor because it has significant side effects, particularly cardiac, and also interacts with other medications with significant potential for harm. While much prescribing on the net is done via reputable doctors and pharmacy chains, much is not, and it is essential that patients do not start taking potentially dangerous drugs because they have used the net as a short cut, often via dubious websites, to obtaining often rather stigmatized treatments.

"B to C", or Business to Consumer, and "B to B", Business to Business, are the two main models of Internet business interaction. Both involve the sale of products, whether they be wheelchairs, paper, medical hardware, information or medications. Whatever the product the Internet is an amazing e-commerce medium, and with the health sector valued at 16% of the USA Gross Domestic Product, there is a lot of value for those who wish to sell health related products. There are many health information sites that only really exist as a disguise, and where the main object of the site is to sell products, often dubious, or useless, to consumers, or health professionals. They often suddenly link you with a range of "natural products" or with sites that encourage spending on a wide range of related products. Even more worrying for the unwary are the sites that send "cookies" (small embedded computer programs) to your computer which can identify your surfing habits, and consequently your interests, to the originating site, so that they may more easily target their sales pitch to you in future. Watch out for the emails full of great ideas for you to spend your money on! Buying health products is like buying anything else – take advice from others, do not spend large amounts of money impulsively, and make sure the product you are buying is of good quality, works effectively and is value for money. Remember that, while you may get great bargains on e-Bay, if you want a product that is guaranteed you will have to go to the manufacturers, or reputable retailers, most of whom now have sales websites anyway.

And now some brief history.

History of the Computer and the Internet

A comprehensive history of computing would have to include the Chinese abacus, Charles Babbage's "analytical engine' of 1834 and the many mechanical calculators built in the nineteenth and early twentieth centuries. However, the first real electronic computer was Turing's "Colossus" used by the British military from 1943 onwards to help break codes used by the German army in World War II. High level programming languages such as FORTRAN were introduced from the mid fifties and the development of integrated circuits and operating systems in the early sixties led to huge gains in computational power and efficacy. In the seventies microcomputers and workstations were introduced as the miniaturization and integration of computer components proceeded. Microsoft was founded in 1975, Apple in 1977 and by 1978 more than half a million computers were being used in the US. The IBM personal computer was introduced in 1981 and the Apple Macintosh in 1984. In 1982 *Time* magazine declared the computer "man of the year." By 1986 the number of computers in the US had risen to over 30 million jumping to 50 million 1989, the year that the first notebook computer appeared. The same year an academic billboard, called the World Wide Web, was invented by Tim Berners-Lee. The last decade has seen an explosion in accessible bandwidth around the world allowing increasingly powerful and flexible computers to interact with each other in real time. In 1993 the first browsers were introduced closely followed by the Internet effectively giving public access to millions. Today there are many thousands of ISPs around the world that service billions of email accounts for today's approximate 1.2 billion Internet users. Traffic on the Internet still doubles every 100 days. This stunning change in the way the world does business was totally unpredicted even 10 years ago.

STRENGTHS AND WEAKNESSES OF THE INTERNET AND EMAIL

These will be comprehensively covered in later chapters, as there are so many clinical issues of significance that are specific to the Internet, especially Internet addictions and phobias. The Internet has gained international acceptance and even countries such as China and Myanmar, which have previously tried to block major sections of the Internet, are beginning to relent. The Internet is widespread and accessible, becoming cheaper, better understood and more user-friendly and flexible with access by satellite to laptops and palm-sized computers, phones and multiple devices embedded in unexpected places, such as cars, business environments, and even our pets, who we now monitor routinely with Global Positioning System software linked to chips embedded under their skin. The recent emergence of the i-phone and blackberry generation of devices, with their extraordinary capacity to download and play music and movies, to act as a phone and messaging system, to use email and scheduling software, and to fully access the Internet for maps, search tools and the like, has simply made the Internet a more accessible and useful tool for use in everyday life.

On the downside the Internet is overloaded and can be a great time waster – no-one can possibly attempt to read all that is available on most common subjects. Remember to always "bookmark" your favorite sites so that you don't spend hours trying to find them the next time you log on.

But perhaps the most annoying thing about the Internet is the way sites come and go. Sites are usually set up by individuals and if they lose interest, don't pay their dues, or simply change their address, the homepage suddenly disappears, usually without a hint as to whether it has moved or died completely. This is particularly evident in the "blogosphere" where online blogs (short for a web log) come and go all the time. For this reason it is always worth checking out any site to find out when it began, and who is responsible for the content. Blogs are difficult to maintain, and many people start them full of enthusiasm, but don't realize how much time it takes to keep them fresh and new to returning callers. Most good blogs take several hours of maintenance and content development each day, and relatively few people have that sort of time to put in to maintaining a site unless they are professional writers or journalists for whom this is a paid role. Think of a blog as being a short online newspaper or journal available 24 by 7, and you will instantly realize how important it is for them to be constantly updated, and monitored, especially as most solicit comments and stories from readers, not all of which are necessarily accurate, publishable, or legally defensible. Be wary of brand new sites that don't seem to have had much thought or effort put into them – they will probably be gone next month! But this weakness is also a strength because the Internet is constantly changing and alive, and good sites are regularly updated to encourage return visits – a good site is usually a "sticky" site - it encourages you to return by constantly offering new content and materials. .

What Evidence is There That eHealth Works?

Actually, not much! Given that most scientifically valid clinical research projects take six months to plan, six months to attract funding and resources, at least a year or more to complete and several months to analyze and write up results before the final wait for publication in a scientific journal, this is hardly surprising. Remember that the Internet is still in it's infancy so the usual research cycle of about 3 years from planning to publication of results has hardly had time to be completed. There are some early evaluations of psychotherapy by email that look positive, but otherwise the Internet is like the phone -everyone just assumes it works but no one has really proved it! There are now several journals that focus on Internet healthcare, notably the Journal of Internet Medical Research (www.jmir.org), which is a reputable peer reviewed general medical journal, and the Internet Journal of Mental Health (www.ispub.com) which is the mental health equivalent. However most of the formal research on Internet healthcare still tends to appear in other medical journals, easily accessible by the general public through PubMed, (http://www.ncbi.nlm.nih.gov/pubmed) the National Institutes of Health academic repository of all peer-reviewed health literature. I have just performed a search using the key words "Internet health outcomes" and from a total of 689 academic papers available that match these search terms the following 7 papers were published in April 2008 alone:

1. Kroeze W, Oenema A, Campbell M, Brug J.
   Comparison of use and appreciation of a print-delivered versus CD-ROM-delivered, computer-tailored intervention targeting saturated fat intake: randomized controlled trial. J Med Internet Res. 2008 Apr 29;10(2):e12.

2. Coiera EW, Vickland V.
   Is relevance relevant? User relevance ratings may not predict the impact of Internet search on decision outcomes. J Am Med Inform Assoc. 2008 Apr 24.

3. Street JM, Braunack-Mayer AJ, Facey K, Ashcroft RE, Hiller JE.
   Virtual community consultation? Using the literature and weblogs to link community perspectives and health technology assessment. Health Expect. 2008 Jun;11(2):189-200. Epub 2008 Apr 22.

4. Wilson C, Flight I, Hart E, Turnbull D, Cole S, Young G.
   Internet access for delivery of health information to South Australians. Aust N Z J Public Health. 2008 Apr;32(2):174-6.

5. Perry M, Draskovi I, van Achterberg T, Borm GF, van Eijken MI, Lucassen P, Vernooij-Dassen MJ, Olde Rikkert MG.

   Can an EASYcare based dementia training programme improve diagnostic assessment and management of dementia by general practitioners and primary care nurses? The design of a randomized controlled trial. BMC Health Serv Res. 2008 Apr 2;8:71.

6. Peña-Purcell N.
Hispanics' use of Internet health information: an exploratory study. J Med Libr Assoc. 2008 Apr;96(2):101-7.

7. Kim J, Ha JS, Jun S, Park TS, Kim H.
The weather watch/warning system for stroke and asthma in South Korea. Int J Environ Health Res. 2008 Apr;18(2):117-27.

Look at the extraordinary variety of research that is being undertaken on Internet healthcare. Just in this quick view it ranges across several countries and cultures, and is as varied as developing weather warning systems, to dementia training programs, to consultation with entire communities. And the two most important papers in this selection are on entirely different topics from these. The first is a randomized controlled clinical trial on nutrition education in the Journal of Internet Medical Research. The second is a paper in the Journal of the American Medical Informatics Association from Enrico Coiera MD, who works in Sydney Australia, and is one of the premier Internet researchers in the world, examining the relevance of key words with respect to search engine outcomes. Internet healthcare is a burgeoning area from a research perspective, but it is still hard for researchers to get funded to do this type of research, as most major funding organizations, such as the NIH, still prefer to fund basic biological research rather than this "applied" form of research.

And one of the reasons there has been so little high quality research and evaluation is the large number of disparate interest groups - all with their own agendas - who are involved in eHealth.

THE PLAYERS

This is where it starts getting complicated - so many groups, each with a high opinion of its own worth and all looking for a bite of the cherry, their share of the profit. These stakeholders cover the gamut of health, education, information technology, finance, defense and social service industries. There are six main groups:

a. Patients and their families, doctors and other health professionals

Mostly these people are united and driven by the simple desire for better quality healthcare. This is the most important group. And with the general acceptance of "consumer driven healthcare" as a national policy direction in most western countries, this group will undoubtedly increase in importance and impact in future. This book is primarily about the relationship between the patient, their doctor and the Internet - by far and away the most important triad in the overall system.

b. Teachers, researchers and students

These are the people who observe and evaluate the process of eHealth. Despite the ubiquity of the Internet, there are still relatively few individuals who call themselves "Internet health researchers" but they are extremely important because their research will demonstrate the effectiveness, or otherwise, of the online care. This research will ensure the therapies are used properly and are funded in the future. The advantage of research on the Internet is that it tends to be relatively cheap to undertake, and there are multiple topics available for examination, but the disadvantage is that it is still a young field of research, and relatively few grants and research funding opportunities are available.

c. Governments, politicians, professional bodies and unions

This is the group that sporadically attempts to regulate and control the development of eHealth. They are also the major funders who need to be convinced of the efficacy of eHealthcare so it can play an even more central role in the provision of health services worldwide. Politicians love e-care systems - as long as they don't have to pay too much for them - because they offer huge possibilities for self-publicity and vote garnering. But there is still enormous ignorance among many in this group, mainly because of their age, and this is perhaps best demonstrated by President George W. Bush's widely quoted comment about "the Internets".

d. Hardware and software developers and retailers

These vary from the profit driven multinationals like Microsoft, Intel and Sun to idealistic individuals who develop software programs or useful clinical gadgets in their homes purely in the hope of helping someone. We couldn't provide any online services without these people but beware the motivations and ruthlessness of the multinationals in particular. There have been many excellent ideas, systems and programs bought by large companies and deliberately sunk without trace to eliminate competition. Why is it that we don't have more agreed standards in healthcare software development, or a national identification number for healthcare? The answer is simple in part – because there is a huge amount of profitable return for investors our current highly inefficient health system that would be reduced if we became more efficient. The mainstream emergence of open source software development over the past decade has been a tremendously positive development which will hopefully eventually lead to the development of standards based open source electronic health records – more about that later.

e. Telephone companies, carriers and Internet providers

These provide the basic infrastructure necessary to carry the online therapies and, again, they are driven by profit. Controlling access to the networks is of critical political importance and the struggle to control this access should not be underestimated. It is fascinating to watch how these companies compete with each other as we gradually move to a world of "mega-corporations" with more and more mergers both between and within separate industrial sectors. Telecommunications companies merging with media outfits. Software companies buying electronic health record service businesses. Hardware manufacturers linking with cable providers. And so it will go on.

f. Lastly - but by no means least - consultants, entrepreneurs and hangers on

Occasionally these people are helpful. But, more often than not, in my experience, they are out for short term financial gains for themselves usually at the expense of the users - patients and clinicians. Beware the "consultant" with generic skills and little useful knowledge, who professes to be an "expert" as a consequence of one previous commercial engagement. Male versions wear dark suits, have greased back hair and are permanently glued to mobile phones. The female version wears stilettos, too much make-up, and constantly flatters her potential employer. If they do win your contract they will invariably recommend that further consultants (themselves) are employed to manage the project in the next stage that they identify! They are drawn, like magpies, to any new and potentially lucrative area such as this, and are best treated with extreme caution and a healthy dose of cynicism!

The development of eHealth involves collaboration between all these different groups. It must be remembered that online systems are simply part of an overall health system. They should not be seen as being ends in themselves but a means to broaden the choices of care available. As long as eHealthcare systems on the Internet are flexible, simple, have built in training, are user friendly, focused on patients' needs and encourage collaborative health efforts, they should be successful. Nobody said it would be easy!

IN SUMMARY:

- The Internet is here to stay and is the largest and most disorganized information source ever known to man

- Over 60% of US Internet users – more than 140 million people – have searched for health information on the Internet

- Patients trust doctors to deliver high quality health information

- There are millions of websites providing health related information on the Internet

- Research on the effectiveness of the Internet in healthcare is still in the early stages

- There are many different players involved in eHealth, and they have very differing motivations.

4

Online Consultations

There are a number of health options on the web for patients. All of these are available now in a variety of forms and will be discussed over the next three chapters. Make sure that your doctor is aware of how you are using the Internet, and ask him or her for advice and assistance. The Internet health options include information provision (for individuals or groups, general or personalized), diagnostic scales or instruments, health risk calculators, support groups (chat or discussion groups, facilitated or not facilitated), expert interactive sessions (live, recorded, video, audio or written), and email access to experts (known or unknown) for consultation. Maybe your doctor is one of these experts, or has access to a number of useful links or tools via their own website.

Let's start with e-consultations. A consultation carried out on-line isn't so very different to one you would have in at your doctor's office or surgery. It should still incorporate:

1. The referral process

2. Gathering information from the patient during the interview and from other people or sources before, during or after the interview

3. Assessing the patient's physical and mental state,

4. Structured questionnaires and assessment tools, and ordering any blood tests or X-rays

5. Confirmation of the diagnosis and prognosis

6 Feedback about the diagnosis, and development of a treatment plan in consultation with the patient, relevant family members and the referrer

These six steps are the traditional ones used in most consultations. In this more modern world an alternative approach that I prefer, is to think of the consultation as having only three phases:

1. Data collection (stages 1, 2 and 4 above)

2. Data Analysis (stages 3 and 5 above)

3. Project Management (stage 6 above)

The advantage of this approach is that it defines more precisely what exactly is going on, and is less mystical than the traditional medical approach, which is more focused on the doctor's process, rather than what is core to the patients needs. It offers more potential involvement for the patient and their family, and I think is simply more straightforward. Of course the success of the whole endeavor ultimately depends on the level of personal and professional trust and commitment between the patient and the doctor. So let's use the more modern approach and see how it integrates the traditional approach, particularly when we are going to be using the Internet as a key component of all three consultation phases.

1. DATA COLLECTION

Usually, the referrer sends information about the patient to the doctor, but not always and many patients, depending on their health insurance, literally walk into a new doctor's office by self-referral with no background information except what they know themselves. Referrals are traditionally sent by letter but increasingly it is by email and, within a few years, it will be sent by video mail. Patients will be video recorded during primary care consultations and the video emailed to the specialist along with any other essential information, such as EKG records and X-rays.

One of the benefits of eHealth is that during this referral period, patients will have the opportunity to find out much more about their doctor through their homepage, or curriculum vitae on the "net." If you cannot find any information about your doctor via Google then I would immediately be somewhat suspicious of their level of experience as almost all experienced doctors nowadays have either their own website or information page, or have been quoted giving a talk at a professional conference or community activity. Of course, this is also a useful source of information for patients having face to face consultations.

Another major benefit for patients is that it is simple for referrers to send copies of referral notes and information to their patients. This is one of the ways that the online healthcare is changing the power balance between doctors and patients.

Traditionally, information is gathered from the patient, the referrer and sometimes family and friends and other health related services. Doctors need:

(a) Basic demographic data – name, age, contact details, next of kin etc

(b) History of present difficulties – symptoms, disability levels, length and extent of problems, previous attempts at treatment

(c) Significant past medical, psychiatric and alcohol and drug use history, present medications and alcohol and drug intake

(d) Family background and history – social and genetic

(e) Personal history including early development, schooling, relationships, work history and any childhood or other traumas

The amount of information collected and the way in which it is collected varies enormously depending on the clinical situation and the requirements of the patient and the doctor. For instance if I am doing an emergency face to face assessment I will often only initially collect information in sections i.-iii above. That may be all that's necessary or possible to collect in a stressful situation and will allow me to make initial diagnostic and treatment decisions. It is not unusual for patients to bring detailed medical histories about themselves to a consultation, and that is generally very helpful. Such histories may include previous letters and results from other doctors, or in some cases are written essays detailing the development of symptoms over long periods of time. I haven't yet had a patient come in and see me with their entire history documented on a website, but I have certainly had a few who have brought in printed copies of word documents that they have created.

Now that we live in the electronic age, referral processes are changing. Where I work, at UC Davis, we have a full electronic medical record, so I am able to access the full medical history of any of our patients referred to me by our primary care physicians. This includes all their notes, results, investigations, operations and background information. I no longer need a referral note from a referring physician as I can literally see the notes they wrote which say "referral to Dr Yellowlees", with the consultation request routed to me electronically.

Other sources of information, such as family, friends or other health agencies, are contacted in exactly the same way for e-care as for face to face consultations. In both situations the patient should be informed of these contacts.

All this information, or medical data, can be gathered either face to face or online. A history taking interview may take a little longer by email, and can be undertaken by phone if speed is of the essence, or even by automated voice response systems. Structured interviews, either written or spoken, can be used to collect the required broad-based information. These are increasingly being used, and many doctors now collect baseline medical data via online questionnaires. After reading this, the doctor can then either ask, or email, more specific questions.

Most of us have filled out some sort of health assessment form at some stage of our lives. These are now widely used in all areas of health to help assess illnesses and disabilities as diverse as impotence, cardiac disease, schizophrenia and arthritis. Questionnaires are well suited to online assessments and are becoming increasingly important to assist with diagnosis and measure treatment outcomes. In my own clinic we use at least half a dozen different questionnaires. Some are very simple while some are long and complicated.

Patients will use questionnaires more and more to monitor their own progress. One of my patients who suffers from depression regularly uses the Beck Depression Scale to check his level of depression. When he comes to see me he brings his weekly rating results to help us measure his progress. Similar questionnaires are available for disorders as diverse as asthma, arthritis, pain, muscle and heart disorders and epilepsy. There are many sites that support self-monitoring designed for parents of children who have Attention Deficit Hyperactivity Disorder. At some of these it is possible to have parents, teachers and doctors all fill in questionnaires so that the doctors can more precisely monitor the various stimulant medications used with these children. This is a much better way of evaluating the effectiveness of these sometimes controversial treatments, and allows the doctor to have much more certainty in prescribing. You can find monitoring questionnaires and tools for virtually any disorder via Google. Go and have a look at them, and then fill them in and discuss the results with your doctor, either online or with printouts.

If you need blood tests, x-rays or any other type of medical investigation, do make sure that you get the results. Traditionally this was a photocopy of a results sheet. Now almost all results are now electronic, and most doctors will be happy to print out copies for you, or give you the results copied to a CD if you take one to your consultation. Of course not all systems allow this to happen unfortunately, but most will in future; after all it is your information. So ask your doctor if you can have electronic copies of any results. Then keep them ideally in a personal health record, if you are one of relatively few people who has these, or at least in an organized electronic file, backed up, on your computer, and of course, on the CD itself as a further backup. You never know when you will need to have copies of results for future consultations. I am sure that there will the development of "health data banks" for such personal information in the not too distant future as we all start collecting longitudinal often personally sensitive data, and don't want to have to transfer all the data every time we buy a new computer. Doesn't it make sense to pay a small amount per year to have our health and probably other important electronic documents secured, just like we pay for a lock box at the bank?

A word here on "Internet therapists" who don't insist on knowing the full name and contact details of their patients and who do not give out their own specific and correct contact details. These "therapists" should be viewed with caution. I do not consider anyone, whatever their training, to be acting professionally if they do not insist on knowing who their patients are. I know some organizations, such as Samaritans, who don't require contact details but as they only deal with crises and don't treat people long term, this is different.

2. DATA ANALYSIS

Data analysis consists of the examination and conclusions drawn from physical and mental state assessments, and the reasoning process that the doctor uses to reach a conclusion about your diagnosis and prognosis. As most of this is dependent on the clinician reviewing information about you, the bulk of this part of the examination should be able to be undertaken online.

Most patients referred for eHealth assessments should also have a physical check up. If you are seeing your doctor face to face as well, and you use eHealth for only some of your consultations, then this is not a problem as any physical examinations required can be done in the normal way when you see your doctor in person. A number of the current online consultation services insist that any patients being treated online have at least an annual physical from a face to face doctor – a very sensible practice.

But what about if you are at some distance from your doctor? At first glance it may seem a tall order to expect online doctors to carry out physical examinations. It's actually not. Experienced doctors base 85% of their medical and psychiatric diagnoses on history alone...with no need for physical examinations, blood screens, X-rays etc. So a great deal of the time your history should be enough for many doctors. And in fact experienced doctors often make their initial hypotheses about the patients diagnosis literally in a couple of minutes, using a combination of experience and unconscious awareness as described in the excellent book, "Blink", by Malcolm Gladwell, the world renowned author of "The Tipping Point". I know that this happens to me all the time when I see patients – and now if I am not reasonably sure of their diagnosis within a few minutes of the interview starting, it means that they are unusual, and in the group of about 10% of patients who are particularly difficult to diagnose.

There are, of course, many occasions when a physical examination is necessary. Well the age of virtual physicals is almost with us. There have now been several studies showing that a nurse performing an examination for which he or she is trained, under the supervision of a doctor observing on a video system, is just as accurate at picking up physical abnormalities as the doctor in the live situation. This is all right when video on the net is available, but most of the time it is not and one has to depend on email. In that situation the best alternatives are to arrange for another local practitioner to do the examination, but to tell them what to look for in particular, or to organize to see the patient yourself.

Digital still or movie cameras are another possibility. These cameras can take pictures of skin lesions, abnormal movements, or close ups of the eye and can then be sent as email attachments. In the same way X-rays, ultrasounds and pathology slides or results can be sent via the Internet from a patient, or doctor, to another doctor or hospital. This is called "store and forward" medicine – in other words some part of the examination is filmed, then stored, and then forwarded to someone else for an opinion. This has been happening in radiology and pathology for many years, and most radiologists and pathologists literally never see patients face to face anymore – they depend completely on information gained from examinations undertaken by others. These store and forward approaches have become widely used in dermatology and ophthalmology in the past few years, especially for skin cancer screening and for screening for diabetic retinopathy.

My prediction is that store and forward techniques will be used in many areas of medicine in future. I am currently undertaking a trial of store and forward psychiatry whereby a colleague interviews patients on camera, writes a structured history I have defined on a website, and uploads about 10 minutes of video clips of significant parts of the interview for me to see. I then review the videos (and here I am using the process described in "Blink" above), read the history, and write an opinion about the patient, which can be seen on the Internet by the referring primary care physician. I undertake a psychiatric examination of a patient I have never met in real time and in the bulk of cases am able to write a treatment plan for the patient's primary provider using clinical guidelines. This consultation takes me only about 20-30 minutes total, in comparison with the 60 minutes it takes for me to see a new patient face to face. Some patients are too complicated or unusual for me to be confident about my opinion in this process, and in those circumstances the patients simply have to travel to be seen – but they would have had to do that anyway had this process not been available, so nothing is lost in those situations. I estimate that about 80-90% of patients will be able to be assessed using this technique, and am undertaking a research program to confirm this. The next stage is to look at what other areas of medicine are compatible with store and forward techniques – probably dementia assessments, many neurological and primary care assessments, and much of pediatrics. What a change in the way we may work in future.

Assessing a patient's mental state is certainly more difficult online than face to face, although with store and forward videos I have been surprised at how relatively straightforward this can be in most instances. Describing someone's mental state is the therapist's equivalent of a physician taking their patient's blood pressure. Assessment procedures are widely taught and practiced in psychiatry, medicine, psychology and nursing in particular, and in my view, should be used by everyone who carries out mental health consultations. After all if a therapist does not attempt to objectively describe the present mental health and behavior of a patient, how are they going to compare them at different points in time to judge the effectiveness of any interventions? And how are they going to describe their patients accurately to their colleagues if required?

There are many different ways of describing a patient's mental state but the following is the assessment guide I use: -

Appearance – the patient's physical presentation, clothing, hygiene and cultural appropriateness

Behavior – the patient's behavioral style, including agitation, slowness, or inappropriate or unusual behavior

Conversation – the content, including direct quotes, and the form of speech, including the rate and logic of the patient's thought processes

Mood – the level and type of mood, its variability, range, appropriateness and intensity

Perceptual abnormalities – symptoms of psychosis or other abnormal phenomena including hallucinations or delusions in any of the five senses of vision, hearing, smell, taste and touch.

Cognition – processes of orientation, memory, attention and concentration

Dangerousness – suicidal or homicidal thoughts, beliefs or feelings

Insight – what the patient believes is their problem, and how realistic this is

Judgment – assessment of the level of judgment, particularly regarding decision making

Rapport – the interaction between the patient and the therapist and, in particular the feelings the patient evokes in the therapist.

This is actually just a simple way of describing anyone. Not all sections have to be completed. Sometimes it isn't possible to complete them all, even in the face to face situation, but even using simple email a large number of these questions can be answered.

There are ways around the problem of a lack of visual cues if video is not available. Patients can provide photographs of themselves, have their relatives or friends give the therapist objective descriptions of them or they can fill out structured interview sheets which contain cognitive tests or questions about their symptoms.

On the other hand, if a face to face assessment can be performed in the first instance, phone and email follow up is much easier, and it is most likely that ultimately many patients will be seen both face to face, and online, depending on convenience and their needs at a particular time. The doctor and patient have got to know each other through the face to face assessment, and the doctor will be more confident of his/her assessment of the patient online as a consequence. A large number of doctors are like me, and have been assessing and treating patients using videoconferencing (or telemedicine) for a number of years. We have learned a lot through this process and are able to transfer our skills to use videoconferencing on the net. Video e- consultations are starting to take off, and increasing numbers of patients are using relatively low cost secure Internet video systems to meet their doctors.

As mentioned previously, data analysis consists of the examination and conclusions drawn from physical and mental state assessments, and the reasoning process that the doctor uses to reach a conclusion about your diagnosis and prognosis.

So what about this reasoning process, and is it any different online, from face to face? Many books have been written about medical reasoning – so much so that it has become virtually a scientific field of study in its own right. This book is not the place for a monologue on medical reasoning, but I do encourage you to read the excellent book by Dr Jerome Groopman MD, entitled "How Doctors Think" if you want a recent review. Suffice to say that good doctors examine all available data as thoroughly as possible; they embrace uncertainty and avoid snap judgments, and use their experience to make sure that they consider a wide range of diagnostic options, which they then narrow down by a logical process of exclusion. My own approach is to constantly ask myself if the data, the history and examination, really "fit" my conclusions, and if my conclusions "feel right", and if they don't I keep on looking until I am satisfied that there is a good match.

In conclusion, to undertake a good diagnostic analysis in the online world, one needs good data. This is one area where the online environment, with electronic health records, and easily accessible electronic blood results and x-rays, for instance, may well lead us to better analyses of patients diagnosis than was possible in a previous face to face world, where often patients were, and still are, assessed with only partial information available to the doctor. I have undertaken many assessments of patients in the face to face world where I knew that there was valuable data available elsewhere, but not accessible to me, and where I have simply had to do my best with limited, and sometimes wrong, information. With online medicine this situation should become less and less common, thank goodness.

3. Project Management

The provision of feedback on the diagnosis and the development of a treatment plan in consultation with the patient, relevant family members and the referrer is really very similar as a process to project management. Here the project is the patient and their illness, the manager is the doctor, the patient and their family, and the outcome is the treatment plan, complete with deliverables (numbers of interventions and appointments), and milestones (timed objective improvements in health outcomes). The project team may involve a large number of multi-disciplinary health professionals, both face to face, and online. What a simple way of looking at the process of care, but how logical, especially when the patient has a straightforward illness that can be treated using a best-practice clinical guideline or self-help process.

Here is where you, as a patient, have a real opportunity to work collaboratively with your doctor, and to use the power of information and the Internet to your advantage. Make sure that your doctor gives you written details of your diagnosis and all aspects of your treatment plan, and ideally a website, or websites, that covers all of these. Then go and do your home work and look everything up. There is a large amount of evidence that proves that the more accurately a patient understands what is happening to them, the more likely they are to do well from a medical viewpoint. If you are feeling too sick, then get your family to look information up for you, and then explain it to you. Ask you doctor any questions you want, and if he or she is prepared to communicate by email, then send a list of questions to them in advance of your next appointment so that you can discuss them when you meet, whether this is face to face or online.

The major advantage of email is that you as the patient have the information in writing and can refer back to it at a later date. This is hugely helpful, not just for the patient, but also for the doctor as a permanent record of exactly what has been "said" to the patient. But one caveat. Don't send multiple short separate questions on email to your doctor – this will fill their inbox and lose you sympathy as it is very hard to respond to lots of separate questions, but much easier to respond to a simple well worked list of queries that follow logically and in sequence. Don't put your doctor off by using online access over-enthusiastically – you have to respect their time, and remember that they have many other patients as well, and quite a number will be in the same situation as you.

Think of yourself as a collaborator in providing care for yourself – and your two main collaborators are your doctor, and the Internet, where the information resides about your project, your illness, your treatment plan. Take advantage of both your collaborators, but be careful not to abuse either of them by over-use.

WHAT CONSULTATIONS ARE AVAILABLE ONLINE?

The short answer is almost any consultations can be performed online! And an increasing number of practitioners are now performing them. Consultations fall into two broad groups - those performed by conventionally and professionally trained practitioners and those undertaken by "alternative practitioners."

A. Conventional clinical practitioners

(i) **Discipline based:** These people are professionally trained in medicine, psychology, nursing or other professional disciplines. It is common for these groups to work in a multidisciplinary manner, each providing specialist input and expertise into the assessment and treatment of individuals with significant medical illnesses. A team approach based on the knowledge and training of individual professionals with overlapping and complementary skills may make these consultations very effective. Patients who email me have almost always seen me face to face previously so my personal use of email for consultations is for follow up, rather than for initial consultations, or when patients cannot get to see me face to face because I am away overseas or in another state, and they want an urgent response to a particular problem. As I know them already I can almost always give them sensible quick advice which saves them having to go to another doctor who doesn't know them as well.

In crisis situations where time is critical telephones are the time-honored solution. Patients with specific problems expect their doctor to help them quickly. To save time the doctor will spend less time exploring the patient's background and more time on the immediate problem and how to resolve it.

Crisis intervention by email can be between doctor and patient or between fellow sufferers, as in the following net example.

Posted by Melancholy guy.

Hey. I'm really at the end of my rope here. Need to hear three things 1. Is it worthwhile trying to keep on realizing yourself when you're down. 2. Somebody out there must know what makes it worth living for. 3. Has real full-blown depression made me lose my centre□□. I'm dead and I'm not even thirty. What I'm depressed over is totally irrelevant to me. I'd rather have cancer than this. I look at people and I can't see their faces. I listen to them but I can't hear what they are saying. Will I ever hear and feel again? If not, what can I expect from life? I'm seeing a psychiatrist but he hasn't prescribed drugs yet. I can't tell him anything relevant about my life. I just feel dead. How can this all be. I'm not even thirty, and I've blown everything. Who can help me?

Reply by Lorna. Shortly after.

Depression is a numbing event. I have my highs and lows. Luckily I have light in my life now. Frustration, no relationships, no job, failure – that's all part of being depressed and living in the social mayhem of the 90's. Whatever the case, have faith in your psychiatrist. A lot of things you mentioned sound like depression talking. You know that body chemistry and psychological aspects of depression are interrelated. If you feel bad physically, stress or something, don't take care of yourself, eat wrong, sleep wrong, and you can wind up feeling tired, irritable and depressed. You get a chem imbalance or something and feel bad physically. Whatever the reason, things will get better. I have been if far worse shape than I am now. I took antidepressants when I was like you. They won't "prove you wrong to yourself" but they can help you gain some perspective while you sort it all out. I am telling you this because #1 there is anonymity here #2 there is hope in this situation. Many many people feel like you do, and you will feel better someday. You will laugh again! Just keep seeing your Doc and don't give up! As you begin to feel better things around you will begin to look better.

B. Alternative practitioners

The most common alternative practices are hypnotherapy, nutritional, orthomolecular, religious and spiritual, yoga and acupuncture.

Many of these therapies are used for stress related disorders and a large number are promoted as working on the mind-body interface. The Internet is a veritable gold-mine for those who are interested in alternative therapies, although, having waded through a large number of sites, many of very dubious quality, I could find none offering consultations by email. There are however a huge number of commercial alternative health sites selling everything from vitamins to light and sound machines to focus on your brain-waves! If you have a yearning to become "qualified" yourself, the "net" offers training in a bewildering array of therapies, usually taking only a few days to complete, and setting you back up to $1,500 a day!

For those who are interested in alternative therapies the National Center for Complementary and Alternative Medicine at the NIH site (http://nccam. nih.gov) is the best place to start. This contains links to a fascinating collection of subjects - look at the types of therapies that come up under just the letter "A" in their collection of therapies to see the breadth of information available:

Actra-Rx
Acupuncture Information
Consensus Statement (NIH Consensus Development Program)
Fibromyalgia treatment (PDF) (Centers for Medicare & Medicaid Services)
Osteoarthritis treatment (PDF) (Centers for Medicare & Medicaid Services)
Aloe Vera: Herbs at a Glance
Androstenedione
Antineoplastons (National Cancer Institute)
(National Cancer Institute)
Aromatherapy and Essential Oils (National Cancer Institute)
Astragalus: Herbs at a Glance
Ayurvedic Interventions for Diabetes (Agency for Healthcare Research and Quality)
Ayurvedic Medicine

And if you want to search more widely around the Internet you can see websites devoted to the following topics as examples of other types of alternative therapies available:

Orthomolecular medicine	Polarity therapy
Naturopathy	Sensory Deprivation

Applied Kinesiology	Biofeedback
Chinese medicine	Gemstone therapy
Homeopathy	Iridology
Macrobiotics	Massage therapy
Music therapy	Breathwork
Hypnotherapy	Yoga
Meditation	Natural hygiene

If these all sound a bit tame, you can also link into the more unusual - such as "urine therapy" for those who fancy drinking their own urine or "trepanation" for those who believe that cutting a hole in the top of their skull is likely to let some light into their lives. I strongly advise against either of these delights!

As with all Internet therapies - be careful! Much of what is available is dubious in the extreme. That is why I strongly advise starting at the NIH website where there is a specific statement indicating that no individual practitioners will be recommended. Think hard before buying anything on these websites and consult with friends, family and your doctor before signing up for any expensive courses, and make sure that you remain in contact with your doctor if you do undertake this style of therapy. If you do decide to, insist on seeing the qualifications and training experience of the therapists. It is quite possible they only have a few days training and are trying to make a profit at your expense.

Important Points to Remember

It is essential patients are assessed as comprehensively online as in a face to face situation. This should be possible in most online situations but does take more effort. It is crucial your doctor or health professional does not to take short-cuts here – that critical decisions are not based on inadequate or inappropriate information.

Information from a variety of sources is especially useful when working online and can usually be easily and rapidly obtained by phone, fax or email. Some Internet sites have tremendous resources and links.

Work with your doctor, and make sure that you use the Internet as a collaborative tool to assist your treatment. Inform your doctor about any information you have found on the Internet. In particular discuss other treatment options you may find, especially if you are undertaking them.

Many patients prefer the extra accessibility and choice that the eHealth offers. I have yet to meet a patient who hasn't wanted more information and choice about their therapeutic options. Gone are the days when the doctor or other therapist patronizingly taps you on the head and says, "There, there, don't worry, I know best." and makes all your health decisions for you.

If I have any doubts at all about the effectiveness of a particular online consultation, arrange a face to face one instead. There is nothing clever about trying to use online technologies exclusively if a face to face consultation is possible and is preferred. This is especially so in an emergency or where someone has an acute illness.

Following the consultation, the doctor should provide written feedback to both the referrer and the patient. I usually send the patient copies of the information I send to the referrer. Consultations are about information exchange and communication and the patient must be central to this process.

Now let's move on to what types of treatment are available online.

5

Treatment And Prevention Online

An amazing fact is that two thirds of the people who use the Internet use it for looking for medical information! 160 million people in the United States alone! And the availability of good quality health information on the Internet means patients can find out more about their problems, sort out their own treatment options. Over the centuries as we have radically changed our minds about the causes of illness, so have our ways of treating it also changed. In 450BC Hippocrates declared that melancholia was caused by excess black bile, and hysteria, by a wandering uterus. Both these ideas remained influential into the 19th Century! At other times in history, depression has been blamed on domination of the soul, gluttony, excessive masturbation, witchcraft, variations in the circulation of the blood, animal spirits and "bad humors." Fortunately treatments have also changed. We no longer burn people at the stake to destroy their inner demons as happened to many thousands of people in the 15th Century.

INFORMATION AGE HEALTHCARE

Dr Richard Smith, past Editor of a British Medical Journal, has talked about the move away from what he called "industrial age medicine" to "information age healthcare". He looked at these two health systems, both in terms of the type of care provided and the cost. Smith has shown how in the medicine of the past, and still as often practiced today, most costs borne by the community are for the actual healthcare system itself, at primary, secondary and tertiary levels. Primary health care includes your family or primary care doctor and community services; Secondary health care is the large number of hospitals around the world; while Tertiary care involves primarily the teaching hospitals in major cities.

With information freely available, consumers having more power, and with the technological and communications revolution, the move to information age health care has become both possible, and increasingly, a reality. Smith saw six levels of care for the future, and these are already emerging. Patients will increasingly be involved in individual self-care at the top, and most important level, particularly in preventing the impact of illnesses. The second level of care involves patients' families and friends, while the third level is essentially networked self-care, such as is increasingly happening through self-help groups, many of which have a significant Internet presence. Professional care is only eventually reached at the fourth level where clinicians, be they doctors or nurses, will act as facilitators, or organizers of care, providing information and analysis of health information for patients to make their own healthcare choices. The next level up is physicians as partners in healthcare, in an equal relationship, working with patients to assist them in the treatment process. Only at the sixth level, where doctors are authorities, does one finally reach what is often thought of as being the traditional "doctor-patient relationship". Here patients turn to doctors for authoritative advice, and allow doctors to make decisions about their healthcare choices. In future we will have to put more and more of our community resources into the levels of self and community care, and less proportionately into formalized health services. This is the information age, where the Internet will increasingly be a crucial healthcare supplement used by doctors and patients alike to ensure good healthcare delivery.

Traditional healthcare treatments fall broadly into three groups:

1. Biological and medically based

2. Educational, social and community based therapies, interventions and prevention programs

3. Self-help and consumer support groups

All these groups use the Internet - at present some more than others but, as patients learn more about the Internet and health care professionals become more flexible, the Internet will become increasingly important for assessment and treatment. But how can you efficiently find the right information about your health from that wonderful disorganized revolutionary medium that we know as the Internet?

SEARCHING THE WEB - A RATIONAL STRATEGY.

It is certainly true that there is a great deal of misinformation on the net, and it is very hard to work out what is good, and what is not. Most people who bring information to me that they have derived from the net tend to have far too much, literally bundles of print outs, and much of it is poor quality. Interestingly more than half of the searches for health information on the web are being performed by partners, carers and loved ones of a sick person, and the single most common reason for Internet searching given by such people is that they are looking for information following the diagnosis of an illness in a loved one. We also know, from the Pew Foundation reports, (www. pewfoundation.org) that most people start searching at a search engines, and then visit many different websites, and that only 27% start their search at a health-related website.

The Internet can be excellent for finding useful information, but you need a sensible search strategy, especially when you are looking for accurate and specific information that will help you make rational decisions, rather than just surfing for fun. I would advise the following four steps as your Internet search strategy, whether you wish to find out what your doctor has published, or what range of treatments are available for asthma. If you are not sure how to use the Internet or perform searches I recommend you do the interactive tutorial course at http://www.netskills.ac.uk/. This is a site run by the University of Newcastle in England that has been providing Internet search teaching since 1995, and now delivers services to all Universities in England. Many other search classes are available via Google, and most libraries offer hands-on classes.

I will cover the four types of searches below. But before you apply these principles I would strongly suggest that for most quick simple searches you go first to www.google.com , and at least scan the first 20 or so results. Just remember that Google displays two types of results, sites ranked by a commercially secret algorithmically derived measure of popularity, which is what most people look at first, and sponsored paid links. Relatively few people go beyond a few pages (40-60) of results from Google, out of the many million that frequently occur. The second place to go routinely is www.wikipedia.com . This open source encyclopedia is just amazing in its breadth and depth. For examples of its extraordinary capacity look at the very comprehensive Wikipedia entries on "Internet search" and "Internet studies" respectively and you will find multiple articles and links of relevance to the topic you are now reading about. The third site to routinely search is www. medlineplus.gov . This is, in my opinion, the best overall consumer health site on the Internet – let me quote the quality guidelines from this site so that you can see why I think this site is so important, and why I recommend it routinely to all my patients.

"MedlinePlus Quality Guidelines

MedlinePlus is designed to help you find appropriate, authoritative health information. To do this, we provide access to information produced by the National Library of Medicine and the National Institutes of Health, such as searches of MEDLINE/PubMed, our database that indexes medical research literature, and ClinicalTrials.gov, the database of research studies from the National Institutes of Health. We also provide you with a database of full-text drug and supplement information, an illustrated medical encyclopedia, a medical dictionary, interactive health tutorials, and the latest health news.

In addition, MedlinePlus contains pages that link to other Web sites. For example, we have Health Topic pages on about 750 diseases and conditions from Alzheimer's Disease to West Nile Virus. We focus on organizing the full-text publications produced by the NIH Institutes and other Federal Government organizations. We also link to other Web sites. The quality guidelines we use in evaluating links to Web pages are listed below.

- Quality, authority and accuracy of health content

  - The organization's mission must relate to the goals of MedlinePlus.

  - The organization must provide accurate, science-based information that complements or enhances the government information found on MedlinePlus.

  - The source of the content is established, respected and dependable. The organization publishes a list of advisory board members or consultants on the site.

  - The information provided is appropriate to the audience level, well-organized and easy to use.

  - MedlinePlus links to original content. MedlinePlus does not link to information reproduced from other Web sites.

  - Lists of links are evaluated/reviewed/quality-filtered.

- The primary purpose of the Web page is educational and not to sell a product or service. Most content is available at no charge.

  - MedlinePlus requires a clear differentiation between content and advertising. There should be an advertising policy on the site. Advertisers or sponsors must not play a role in selecting or editing health information.

  - MedlinePlus will exclude organizations and Web resources if presentation or content could lead a reasonable user to infer endorsement of products or services.

  - MedlinePlus provides links to directories to help you find health professionals, services, and facilities. NLM does not endorse or recommend the organizations that produce these directories, or the individuals or organizations that are included in the directories.

- Availability and maintenance of the Web page

  - The Web site is consistently available.

  - The Web site maintains its links to outside sources.

  - Links from the site are maintained.

  - The source for the contents of the Web page(s) and the entity responsible for maintaining the Web site (webmaster, organization, creator of the content) is clear.

  - Information is current or an update date is included.

  - Registration is not required to view the information on the site.

- Special features

  - The site provides unique information to the topic with a minimum of redundancy and overlap between resources.

  - The site contains special features such as graphics/diagrams, glossary, or other unique information.

  - The content of the site is accessible to persons with disabilities."

This is a very comprehensive description of why the information on www.medlineplus.gov can be trusted. My advice is to bookmark this site as one of your favorites and keep using it.

Now lets move on to the four broad categories of searches that I recommend if you need more comprehensive or in-depth health information:

1. Professional journal searching

There are several free programs on the Internet which will allow you to search professional scientific papers from the health and medical journals. You might as well learn to search in the same way your doctor will - all of the scientific papers quoted in these databases will have been peer-reviewed. The two main professional databases are:

"Medline" (http://www.ncbi.nlm.nih.gov/PUBMED at the NIH and

"Psycinfo" (http://www.apa.org/psycinfo/ at the American Psychological Association

Medline is the premier library search engine that reviews all important peer-reviewed medical journals. This is almost always where your doctor will look first. I do several Medline (also called pubmed) searches every week on average. That a journal is "peer-reviewed" is important. All papers in the journal will have been reviewed by experts who often suggest significant changes or improvements before publication. Many peer-review journals only publish fifteen to twenty percent of papers they receive so their standard is extremely high. Medline started in 1955 and is run from the NIH, and from 2008 onwards full text articles of all papers published about research that has been funded by the NIH will be available via this database. Up until now such articles are often only available online as short abstracts, with the publishing journals charging for individual copies. At present Medline is searched about 70-80 million times every month – so when you do a search here, you won't be alone! While you are looking at pubmed, travel around the site and discover the many databases of genomic data, books, data-mining and visualization tools, and, amazingly, take a look at the components of the human genome that have been fully uncovered and which are shown on the site. This is a real look at the future of personalized medicine, where doctors will check out your genetic code, as well as your chemistry, and prescribe the drug that best suits your overall molecular makeup. This form of medicine is coming soon.

Psycinfo is published by the American Psychological Association and is the premier psychological database search engine. It is not as large as Medline but still has over 2.5 million articles from 1800 onwards, adding about 10,000 papers per month as it covers the scientific contents of over 2100 journals in 49 countries and 27 different languages. PsychInfo also covers a large number of books, and degree dissertations, making it much broader in content area than other databases.

Getting the information you need from both Medline and Psycinfo is easy. First put in the topic of your search, eg arthritis. The search engine then gives you the number of papers which contain that word - in this case far too many! If you wish to make the search more specific, add extra keywords which will reduce the number of papers you get. Generally, it is best to start off with a broad general word such as arthritis and then narrow down the search …eg arthritis followed by treatment-males-outcomes. You would then get copies of all papers related to the treatment outcome of arthritis for males. Both websites offer instructions on how to search, so spend a few minutes reviewing these and you will get much better results for your effort.

To obtain background on your doctor make sure you search on different variations of their name to find all their publications. For example my scientific papers have been published under "Peter Yellowlees", "PM Yellowlees" and "P Yellowlees" and search engines won't fully discriminate between these different versions of the same name. If you just put "Yellowlees" into the engine you will find all of my papers, but also a surprising number of other papers from other members of my family, and some people with the same unusual name that I have only heard of through the Internet! If you want to know more about your doctor then combine a pubmed search, with some time on Google, and between the two approaches you should find most of the available information written by them, or about them. And of course if you do a Google image search you may well find photographs of them, and see what interests they have.

2. Search evaluated Internet subject gateways

There are a number of health sites that have been specifically set up to provide high quality health information for patients and professionals - in the jargon of the Internet these are now called "evaluated gateways." These sites attempt to ensure quality information by either using their own experts, or linking only with other sites whose information they have carefully assessed, or who have an acknowledged level of expertise in the area - major University sites are an example. They are also generally independent and run either by government agencies or consumer organizations, do not take paid advertisements, and have effective quality mechanisms in place to ensure that biased information is less likely to occur.

The beauty of Internet searches is that you can pick up useful reliable information which hasn't been published in peer-reviewed journals. The gateways I use are the US National Library of Medicine (http://locatorplus.gov) or Healthfinder (www.healthfinder.gov) in the US, or Intute (http://www.intute.ac.uk) or NHSDirect (www.nhsdirect.nhs.uk) in the UK. Other sites offer ways of evaluating the quality of patient information (www.discern.org.uk) while some are devoted to collecting peer-reviewed "best practice" treatment guidelines (www.guideline.gov) which you can use to compare with your own treatment regime. If your doctor doesn't know about these sites please tell them! If you want information on evidence-based medicine you cannot go past the Cochrane Library (www.cochrane.org).

I tend to be wary of most commercial health sites, although WebMD (www.webmd.com) is an exception. The main site has well written helpful information primarily focused on patients, and is most certainly worth regular visits. WebMD sponsors two sister sites run in parallel to the main site, both mainly targeting health professionals. These are eMedicine (www.eMedicine.com) and the Medscape Journal of Medicine. (www.medscape.com). Both are excellent peer-reviewed high quality resources that I personally use all the time, and to which I am a contributor. eMedicine describes itself as the original open access comprehensive medical textbook for all clinical fields with currently 6,500 articles from over 10,000 contributors. If you want a detailed review of a topic this is an excellent place to visit. I regularly print out review papers from this site for patients, and use them to discuss the various treatment options available. The Medscape Journal of Medicine is the first online journal to be fully indexed on Medline, and is edited by George Lundberg, MD, the very influential and well known ex-editor of the Journal of the American Medical Association. Many of the peer-reviewed articles, especially the editorials, on this site are presented as both video and written materials, with the authors professionally filmed presenting their work. These video academic presentations are surely the way of the future, and are much more interesting to "watch" than the traditional method of reading. It is also really good to see the author, as this gives the "reader" a better idea of the type of person they are.

You will probably find that you may well go to the gateways before doing a database Medline search because these are still reliable sources, and tend to have more systematically presented information that often summarizes areas of interest, whereas Medline picks mainly scientific papers which are usually much narrower in their content. Take your pick.

3. Web searches

Now we move to the web itself. Here you will have to start questioning the quality of the information you retrieve much more critically as most of it will not have been subjected to any real quality review mechanism, and much will have a commercial bias. It is certainly worthwhile doing though. There are numerous search engines on the web, and they all serve the same functions. They attempt to find as much specific information as you request, as easily as possible. But of course they are all different, use different search approaches, and cover different sets of sites. For a detailed list of the many hundred search engines available just go to wikipedia.com

I mainly use two such engines when looking for health related information for patients on websites around the world, Google and Yahoo. Google (www.google.com) is huge and indexes billions of pages. Without doubt it is the "big daddy" of the search engine industry and has a number of excellent ways of searching for different types of material, and for advanced searching. I strongly suggest that you spend some time on Google clicking around all the different search options and trying them out – don't just stick with the basic search screen. You will find that the advanced searches really do give you much more specific information. There are only two caveats with Google. Firstly no-one outside the company really knows the algorithms they use to rank order search returns, so you certainly cannot guarantee that the first website on your search is the "best" – more likely is the most commonly accessed, and with the "viral marketing" approaches used on the Internet, this may still mean that the top site has biased or inaccurate content. Secondly, sponsors pay for links on Google by buying preferences for certain key search topics or words that will then statistically make their own websites appear high on the list of sponsored links – the more words you buy, and the more you pay, the more likely your website is to appear in the sponsored list. There is of course nothing wrong with this, and I do this to advertise the UC Davis Informatics Program for instance, but as a user you simply need to be aware of the process used to develop the sponsored links.

Yahoo (www.yahoo.com) is Google's main competitor, and also has an excellent search engine, with a particular emphasis on consumer information, and a well set out strategy for defining your question more accurately. There are many more sites listed in Wikipedia, and of course you can always go to the various commercial health portals whose main strength is their immediacy, and ability to bring you up to date health information from all sorts of sources. Consider also subscribing to their electronic newspapers especially if they can send you only news stories that match search criteria that you have defined.

Try doing some Internet searches on your online or face to face doctors as the information you'll find on the Internet will probably be very different to what you glean from a journal search. The Internet search may turn up some of the same academic papers but you may also find them on other websites -

maybe they play in a rock group or on a sports team. They could easily have their own website. Their curriculum vitae might be available online. All this information will give them a human face and give you a pretty good idea of their professional life and their personal interests and motivations to help you to decide whether they are right for you.

If, in 2008, your doctor is not featured somewhere on the Internet at least with a brief summary of their background, then, unless they are still in, or relatively recently out of, a residency program, the alarm bells should be sounding.

4. Check out discussion lists and newsgroups

The final part of your strategy is the one where you can waste most time, and where information is least reliable - but it can be fun, and is sometimes helpful. You may be lucky and join a group where there is a real expert who can answer your precise questions. To find groups go to Google groups (http://groups.google.com/group/HealthyLiving) where the site summarizes its aim as follows:

"Share information on Healthy Living - nutrition; exposing lies re: food; exposing drugs & chemicals; conflict/interest in gov't; exposing lies re: AIDS & other diseases;.Vits; Minerals; amalgam fillings; aspartame; fluoride; GM food; vaccine dangers more. Not for advertising your product or services."

Certainly if you have a very specific question that is somewhat unusual then it is well worth "putting out the word" to relevant lists - you will hit gold surprisingly often. In your bookshop, or an online retailer like Amazon or Barnes and Noble or bookfinder.com, it is not too difficult to find books that have been written describing multiple lists and discussion groups as well. If you use the search terms "Internet health sites" you will find large numbers of books appear recommending multiple websites.

Do be careful with discussion lists and chat rooms - there are some very misleading people out there, and I know of examples where patients have been put off having the best medical treatment available, particularly for cancer, because they have been given wrong or potentially dangerous information in a chat room. Dr Gary Doolittle, an excellent oncologist from Kansas with years of experience in telemedicine, who also encourages his patients to email him, has seen this happen on several occasions, and has had to spend quite a lot of time providing accurate information to previously misinformed patients in order to let them make the best choice about their cancer therapy. I suggest you treat information you get in chat rooms with the same degree of critical skepticism that you would of information gained in a casual conversation with people you have only just met at a social function. And in particular remember that this is where a number of predators "hang out" looking for child victims, as demonstrated by the MSNBC program "to catch a predator" hosted by Chris Hansen, which regularly catches Internet pedophiles and turns them over to the police. So if your children are spending lots of time in chat rooms, my advice to you is simple, stop them.

Now that you know how to search the Internet in a rational and organized manner let's look at the types of treatments on offer.

BIOLOGICAL AND MEDICALLY BASED THERAPIES

Most illnesses have a basic biological cause, often genetically related, and may be triggered by physical or psychological stress. Stresses include psychological traumas such as rape, social distress such as unemployment and physical stress caused by accidents, head injuries and alcohol or drug abuse. Most illnesses are treated with a combination of medications as well as by educating patients and their families.

Both approaches to treatment may occur online. It is well known that doctors base 85-90% of their diagnoses on a patient's history alone so, as long as the doctor or therapist is able to make a good detailed assessment, treatment can be effectively carried out by video, email or phone. The following case study is an example of combination treatments using several technologies, practitioners and therapeutic modalities.

Joan is a 51 year old farmer's wife living on an isolated rural community. Her last child moved away to the city to find work, she suffered from chronic back pain from years of heavy lifting around the farm and she was constantly lonely. Her husband worked long hours on the farm and was constantly irritable, tired and worried about finances. The future looked bleak. None of the children wanted to take over the farm and a property slump meant selling it was not an option. She was depressed and in constant pain.

Joan was examined by an internist using telemedicine at her local clinic. She was diagnosed as having a severe arthritis and major depression and was given an explanation of her disorders. Further information was provided through an Internet mental health site run by a pain support group. The clinic nurse kept in close touch with her by phone and fax and made occasional visits, helping her with some simple cognitive techniques to improve her mood and cope better with her pain. Her primary care physician reviewed her every two weeks, and her treatment program, involving regular painkillers and antidepressants, which involved her husband, was overseen by a psychiatrist who reviewed her by telemedicine every couple of months, and who she was able to contact by email on a weekly basis. She gradually improved and after a year was taken off the antidepressants. She continued to keep in close contact with the clinic nurse who had become as much a friend as a therapist.

There are many online pharmacies on the net. It is possible for you to obtain a prescription from a doctor online, order your medication from the online pharmacy and even have them delivered to your door. But make sure your doctor knows what you are doing and what medication you are taking! There are a lot of important practical and ethical issues involved here, and these will be dealt with later.

Multinational pharmaceutical companies are now dovetailing the release of new drugs with the formation of 24 hour telephone centers staffed by nurses to provide advice and information on these new drugs. The patient's doctor is also notified by fax or email of any inquiries from their patients so they may follow up if necessary. The companies also directly market to patients via television and the Internet, often offering cheap or free starter medication packs – again raising many ethical and practical issues. This is an area that is going to be increasingly important in future as direct to patient marketing will undoubtedly increase.

EDUCATIONAL, PSYCHOLOGICAL, SOCIAL AND COMMUNITY FOCUSED THERAPIES AND INTERVENTIONS AND PREVENTION PROGRAMS

Prevention is always better than cure. There are many ways to prevent illness - mostly through community education and behavioral change leading to more immunizations, better ante-natal care and better nutrition for example. In the first ten to fifteen years of our lives we have the ability to soak up masses of information. This is when many of our lifelong habits are formed. Although there are some preventive health programs for young children and adolescents, most are poorly thought out, taught by non-experts and are often not easy to access, and they tend to be poorly funded and are frequently the first target of cuts if health budgets are reduced. Knowledge about healthy relationships and lifestyles is mostly seen as less important than the traditional "3 R's" – Reading, Riting and Rithmatic! We know that certain types of behaviors are risky and that some occupational groups tend to be more affected by certain disorders than others. Doctors are a good example. Many doctors abuse alcohol and drugs, have marriage problems and have a higher than average rate of suicide. They tend to be hard working focused individuals who often put work before outside interests. They manage their own stress badly while continuing to help others.

The sad thing is that although we know how to prevent these disorders we've have never got around to doing much about it. The advent of online technology is changing this and over the next few years will have an enormous impact in delivering prevention strategies.

How Online Technology Will Help Prevent Illness

Pregnant women can now be screened and their pregnancies monitored more effectively. If they or their children are at high genetic, social, or medical risk they can be given special attention, the children followed up more closely and comparisons made using case registers - large collections of data held online from similarly affected children - to detect any developmental abnormalities as soon as possible. Online education about healthy eating and exercise during pregnancy is available and many women are now monitored by both their obstetrician and their primary care physician in a process of "shared care" that increasingly requires the exchange and sharing of electronic medical information.

My daughter in law has just gone through a pregnancy that has involved her spending a lot of time on the Internet – checking her health records, looking at her baby's ultrasounds posted on youtube.com, monitoring her physical and psychological health by comparing herself against expected milestones, reading and learning about all aspects of pregnancy, and perhaps most importantly contacting and chatting with other pregnant women to support each other. Our son, on the other hand, has been busily buying many of the materials they need for the new baby from Internet sources, including setting up their baby shower lists online. How the Internet has changed pregnancy.

Mass education on health is needed to prevent illnesses and some countries are now getting serious about this. Malaysia has four eHealth projects in the pipeline - one a massive public health education program, with online outlets planned all over the country. Similarly Singapore plans on making the Internet accessible to all citizens and England has set up massive educational programs via the National Health System.

The various talking therapies are, of course, ideal for the Internet. Take a trip to psychcentral.com if you want to see a reputable site that offers access to multiple online therapists, and where many online discussion groups are hosted. If you can provide psychotherapy by letter, as used to be the case, then it is certainly possible via the Internet, and even more so as the multiple communications technologies coalesce and become more powerful.

Cognitive-behavioral psychotherapy, or CBT, is the "thinking and doing" approach to therapy. The cognitive, or "thinking", component assumes that we develop certain set patterns of thoughts which we then act on consciously or unconsciously. Hence if we think in negative patterns we get negative outcomes and may become depressed. The therapeutic task is to confront the negative thoughts and replace them with a more positive set to gradually relieve the depression. The "doing", or behavioral, component is like training an athlete to improve their performance - the anxious person who hyperventilates is taught to control their breathing and relax; the alcoholic is taught to reduce their drinking by avoiding stimuli that have led to drinking in the past. The asthmatic is taught to differentiate between shortness of breath caused by asthma, and that caused by anxiety.

Many online computer programs to treat many anxiety and phobic disorders are now available – for some really good examples have a look at www.moodgym.anu.edu.au. Moodgym is a program developed by Dr Helen Christensen at the University of Canberra in Australia, and which has now been used with over 200,000 patients. Some programs still require a therapist to be present at least part of the time, but some, often designed like multimedia games, can be used by patients on their own. By reacting to cues given during a telephone or computer conducted interview, patients assess their own condition at home, and can undertake a supervised online treatment program.

At a more mundane level important personal experiences of Internet psychotherapy are now becoming available. The following was published at www.metanoia.org, and is now hosted at psychcentral.com

" I am fairly knowledgeable about psychotherapy (for a lay person) and was fortunate to work with a very talented psychotherapist for several years, experiencing the full depth and richness of that experience. I also had the experience of corresponding by email with another psychotherapist over a period of about six months. I experienced deep emotions while reading and writing – grief, anxiety, joy, love, rage, you name it – and explored some very deep issues. I learned to trust and depend on this person. The therapist was usually able to sense my feelings from changes in my writing. Transference happened. The relationship was reflected in my dreams. I was challenged, comforted and empowered. The experience was profoundly healing, and my life changed for the better."

This description shows it is possible to have a deep and therapeutic relationship by email. If we accept that the relationship or bond is the main healing factor in most dynamic psychotherapies, then psychotherapy by email must be possible. The increasing numbers of people falling in love on the Internet is further proof that deep relationships are possible online. If you still doubt this, then think of books and literature - the power of the written word. Throughout history relationships have been maintained and enhanced through letter writing. Perhaps it has happened to you. Think of the authors that you love, whose writing styles you adore. Even though you've never met them you form relationships with them through their books. If one day you do meet them…. maybe you go to their lecture… you'll usually compare them with the perception you have built up of them.

Even group therapy is available on the net. Yvette Colon, an experienced social worker, facilitated some early therapeutic groups in an online community called Echo. It gave her a fascinating insight into the dynamics of group therapy online.

"Online groups, depending on how they are structured, can offer an immediate feeling of safety that makes members feel comfortable. This can allow members to achieve closeness at a safe distance, resulting in their feeling less inhibited to examine aspects of themselves or issues that they might hesitate to explore in a face to face group. Increased self-disclosure and bonding can occur earlier in the online group process than in a traditional group, and this blurs marks of difference like race, culture and sexuality."

It will be fascinating to see where online dynamic psychotherapy leads. Dr Ellen Rothchild, MD wrote *"psychotherapy by letter is nothing new; Freud analyzed "Little Hans" this way."* He also conducted his own self-analysis with *Fliess by letter. Perhaps it's a shame that Freud is no longer alive - he would have loved the opportunity to use online technologies!".*

There have now been some formal research studies undertaken on Internet group therapy, and they are starting to have positive results. One such study published showed significant improvements over the course of a year following hospitalization for a group involved in regular facilitated meetings in a chat room, compared with a control group. Several academic books on all types of Internet therapy, individual and group, including a very comprehensive review edited by Adam Joinson and his colleagues from Oxford, England, and another by Marlene Maheu and her colleagues in the USA, are now available.

Having said all this it's important to remember that psychotherapy by email is more difficult, may take longer and is not generally preferred if it is possible for you to see your doctor face to face. Online psychotherapy is generally more tiring for therapists than face to face. Talking to a screen or typing solidly for several hours to a series of patients is more strenuous than seeing patients in the office. And it's not much fun staring at a computer or TV screen all day!

VIRTUAL REALITY THERAPY

The ultimate form of online CBT is "virtual reality therapy." By simply wrapping on your surround sound and vision multimedia headset you can be instantly transported to a cliff edge, soaring in a plane thousands of feet above the ground or simply surrounded by a gathering of thousands of spiders - depending on your phobia.

The phrase "virtual reality" was coined by Jaron Lanier in 1989 to describe computer simulations of physical environments. Since the mid-1990s, the video game industry and 3D graphics card manufacturers have driven forward the state of personal computer graphics, advancing it far beyond the needs of most business users. These systems range in capability from simple displays of 3D objects to entire virtual cities. Virtual reality systems are now being routinely implemented on personal computers for a variety of activities. One of the most popular virtual reality programs is Second Life, produced by Linden Lab, Inc. Second Life is a general-purpose virtual world accessible through any Internet-connected personal computer. In order to interact in Second Life, users create "avatars", or animated characters, to represent themselves. Individuals use these avatars to maneuver through various "worlds", complete with buildings, geographical features, and other avatars. While the system borrows heavily from video game technology, it is not a game – there are no points, no levels, no missions, and nothing to win. It is simply a platform by which people can create virtual communities, model geological, meteorological, or behavioral phenomena, or rehearse events. And I have been working in Second Life for several years now.

Users of Second Life include a variety of education organizations, from Harvard Law School to the American Cancer Society. There are currently areas of the virtual world that provide such disparate services as teaching heart sounds and auscultation technique, providing social support for individuals with Asperger's Syndrome, and modeling the effects of tsunami on coastal towns. The system has over 8 million account holders from all over the world, most of them with free basic accounts. Approximately 800,000 of those users are active, with over 80,000 of them connected to the system at any time. Virtual reality programs such as Second Life are increasingly being used for educational purposes in a variety of fields, including medical training and disaster preparedness. Linden Lab currently operates the Second Life Education Wiki (http://www.simteach.com/wiki/index.php?title=Second Life Education Wiki), which functions as a source of information for educators and trainers in a variety of fields who wish to use Second Life for distance learning or large-scale training purposes. A number of government agencies, including the Department of Homeland Security, the Centers for

Disease Control, the National Institutes of Health, and the National Science Foundation, have begun using Second Life to hold meetings, conduct training sessions, and explore ways to make access to information more readily available around the world. A recent comprehensive survey intended to gather information on the activities, attitudes, and interests of educators active in Second Life conducted by New Media Consortium reported that the majority used it for educational purposes such as teaching and taking classes as well as for faculty training and development.

VIRTUAL REALITY IN MEDICINE

Virtual reality techniques, involving three-dimensional imaging and surround sound, are increasingly being used in diagnosis, treatment, and medical education. Initial applications of virtual reality in medicine involved visualization of the complex data sets generated by computed tomography (CT) and magnetic resonance imaging (MRI) scans. A recent application of these techniques for diagnostic purposes has been "virtual colonoscopy," in which data from a contrast-enhanced abdominal CT scan is used to make a "fly-through" of the colon. Radiologists then use this fly-through for colon cancer screening. Recent improvements in methodology have brought the sensitivity and specificity of this technique nearly to the levels of optical colonoscopy, and patients prefer the technique to the traditional method.

Virtual reality has also been used extensively to treat phobias (e.g., fear of heights, flying and spiders) and post-traumatic stress disorder. This type of therapy has been shown to be effective in the academic setting, and several commercial entities now offer it to patients (http://www.virtuallybetter.com; http://www.vrphobia.com). In one of my projects we have used a virtual psychosis environment to teach medical students about the auditory and visual hallucinations suffered by patients with schizophrenia.

Virtual reality has been used to provide medical education about healthcare responses to emergencies such as earthquakes, plane crashes and fires. While the primary advantage in phobia treatment is a "safe environment" which patients can explore, the primary advantage in emergency preparedness is simulation of events that are either too rare or too dangerous for effective real-world training. The immersive nature of the virtual reality experience helps to recreate the sense of urgency or panic associated with these events.

Virtual reality programs have also been used for a variety of medical emergency, mass casualty, and disaster response training sessions for medical and public health professionals. One study developed a protocol for training physicians to treat victims of chemical-origin mass casualties as well as victims of biological agents using simulated patients. Although it was found that using standardized patients for such training was more realistic, the computer-based simulations afforded advantages over the live training, such as increased cost effectiveness, the opportunity to conduct the same training sessions over and over to improve skills, the ability to use "just-in-time" learning techniques and experience the training session at any time and location, and adjusting the type and level of expertise required to use the training for various emergency response professionals. Another group of investigators explored the potential for training emergency responders for major health emergencies using virtual reality. Their objective was to increase exposure to life-like emergency situations to improve decision-making and performance and reduce psychological distress in a real health emergency.

Experience with recent natural disasters and terrorist acts has shown that good communication and coordination between responders is vital to an effective response. In my work with Sacramento County, in California, in developing a virtual mass disaster emergency clinic to hand out antibiotics to the population following a massive anthrax bioterrorism attack we have found important advantages of the virtual world, over the real world, for training first responders.

Responders to such events come from many different organizations, including fire, police, military, and hospital personnel. There are three major difficulties in training and evaluating these first responders in the real world:

1. They have little or no chance to train together before the event occurs and hence lack teamwork skills.

2. What training they may have had comes at great cost, in large part due to the effort and need to transport so many people to a specific training site at a specific time.

3. The training sites frequently cannot be the most common targets – for example, one cannot shut down the Golden Gate Bridge during rush hour to train for an earthquake or terror scenario.

Virtual reality offers some intriguing advantages over the real world for these aspects of first responder training, as all of the above difficulties can be overcome. Virtual reality systems can support multiple simultaneous users, each connecting to the system using standard office personal computers and ordinary DSL or cable modem Internet access. Lifelike models of buildings, roads, bridges, and other natural and man-made structures where the users can interact can be constructed. Finally, the whole scenario can be digitally preserved and a full workflow analysis can be performed retrospectively. Public health officials and first-responders can work through the scenarios as many times as they like to familiarize themselves with the workflow and emergency protocols, without encumbering the time and expense of organizing a mock emergency in real life.

Virtual Reality treatments are rapidly becoming more available. They are currently being used to treat post-traumatic stress disorders caused by wartime experiences, and US servicemen are now increasingly being offered such programs. Rather than the traditional method of confronting old nightmares, online technology is able to deliver treatment in a far more therapeutic and humane way. Patients are "transported" to the battlefront and fears and traumas are resolved in virtual place and real time. Virtual Reality is here to stay, and will increasingly be used widely in a number of areas of healthcare.

SELF HELP AND CONSUMER FOCUSED GROUPS AND THERAPIES

The Internet is home to an extraordinary number and variety of online groups and self-help or support programs - many owned and run by patients for their own special needs. Some groups are obviously therapeutic, sometimes set up or mediated, by health professionals. They exist as mailing lists or news groups, where meetings are spread over periods of days – asynchronous meetings. Or they may be real time conferences or chats using synchronous communication. The single main advantage of "cyberspace" for patients and doctors or therapists, is that people with similar interests and concerns can meet each other easily.

Posted by Andrea in response to a question about what was good and bad about online.

I like the online forum because it gives us the chance to talk things through without hurting friends or family. If I said some of the things I have said here to my boyfriend, for example, I know he would misinterpret me and not be objective. Here I can get some support from people who just want to help rather than because they have an ulterior motive in seeing me act in a certain way. Sometimes we just need someone to listen and if we give out to those around us it make them really upset or angry. If I rabbit on and on here then I feel no one is going to reply to me unless they really want to. It helps me a lot because I'm not troubled enough to be on meds or anything, but I do get depressive episodes which I find difficult to deal with. And sometimes we can really make someone feel better without even knowing their full name!!

People are finding that on the 'net' there is always someone to listen and give support in a safe and anonymous environment. Some examples in a 'netshell':

On alcohol

Posted by Dodo:

SHIT!!! I've been grogging on for years to ease my anxiety. I'm in a vicious cycle – on a downward spiral. The alcohol doesn't work – it's just a temporary sedative that wears off. Your problems bounce back. I've drunk so much that I'm addicted to the F☐☐. stuff. I'm in danger. No f☐☐.doctor will give me any meds to dope me up. I'd rather take them than booze. Anyone else the same?
Reply by Cas.

I'm 33 and have been addicted to alcohol for 20 years. I quit drinking 3 ½ years ago but started up again ½ year ago. It was the most foolish thing I ever did. When I was in my 20's I played in a traveling rock band and drank so much (constantly) I was having D.T's by the time I was 26 (convulsions – audio/visual hallucinations, delerium☐.) I also have had panics and anxiety for about as long as the booze which always made it worse (when I started drinking the next morning which I usually did). To cut a long story short I quit drinking for good on April 30ᵗʰ and will never drink again for as long as I live. I take more pills than my shrink likes but now take them to feel normal, not to be cooked. I used info at a website to keep me rational and will send details.

On obesity

Posted by Obscene.

Does anyone else eat and eat, continuing to destroy themselves? At 253 pounds I wake up every morning and say "this is the day I will do it!!". And every day I fail. Every day I look in the mirror and I am stunned at how much weight I have gained. Sometimes I don't even recognize myself. I hate the way I look and yet I love the comfort of food. I'm terrified of feeling hungry. I wish I could unzip some great zipper and step out of my fat self. Tonight has been especially bad – I have eaten soooo much. I feel so sad, alone and fat.
Reply by Jennifer

Yes! I always loved my food, but had been keeping things mostly under control until my older daughter committed suicide in June 1995. After that I seriously overdid it on food, and ended up gaining 60 pounds (and I'm short so it looks a lot more). I am currently battling with Food Problem by switching to lower-fat foods and exercising almost every day. The weight is coming off slowly. I've also got help getting over my daughter's death and that has helped me control my urge to eat whenever I feel sad. Try making small practical goals, like "today I will walk around the block" instead of "from this moment on I will be perfect".
Reply by Carrie

I had to mail you right away because I know exactly how you feel. I used to weigh 210 pounds and loved chocolate. Do females buy more chocolate than males? I've found out that there are no bad foods – you just have to modify the amount. I still eat chocolate and ice cream, but now I am addicted to exercise rather than food. It was difficult changing and I only started with walking half an hour three times per week. I now walk the dog for an hour each day, do weights three times per week, biking, aerobics and rollerblading. It's all possible. Hang in there and keep some positive thoughts – I know you can do it.

While these examples are uplifting, as in everything there are potential downsides, and in the case of the Internet one of these is junk email, now more commonly called "spam".

DEALING WITH SPAM

Spam is junk email, and is a real curse. If you want a good review of all the different types of spam go to wikipedia.com and read their comprehensive listings. As a doctor who practices eHealth I receive chain letters, invitations to pornographic sites and direct pitches for various products literally by the hundreds every day, but luckily the University's sophisticated email filter cuts out most of these from my immediate inbox. It's a real problem for people whose email address is widely known. It is intrusive and personally disturbing. If it is coordinated in a malicious manner it can even be used to completely block and destroy your server, website and email account, in what is now called a "denial of service" attack. This is cyberspamming.

The speed and ease of email means that literally hundreds of thousands of direct mailings can be sent at the touch of a button. Recipients of these unsolicited mailings can feel vulnerable and exposed. Who knows your address? How did they get it? Who is it being passed on to? How will they use it? What is going to turn up in the email next?

Each time you log on to a chatline, to a newsgroup, or even to some homepages, your personal email address can be grabbed. Your rights to privacy are endangered as you address is added to thousands of others, and then unscrupulously sold to companies with the ethical principles of a sewer-rat in a cesspit. It has been estimated spammers reap US$0.003c for each filched email address they sell to commercial "sales" lists – that's US$300 for every 10 million addresses. Unfortunately in this "industry" it is hard to really define the commercial values and profits made. It's hardly surprising we receive uninvited junk email! And look at the countries that spam comes from. Sadly a 2007 study showed that over a quarter of all Internet spam starts in the USA. Here is the list of the "top" or most offending countries where spam is concerned.

1. USA - 28.4%;

2. South Korea - 5.2%;

3. China (including Hong Kong) - 4.9%;

4. Russia - 4.4%;

5. Brazil - 3.7%;

6. France - 3.6%;

7. Germany - 3.4%;

8. Turkey - 3.0%;

9. Poland - 2.7%;

10. Great Britain - 2.4%;

11. Romania - 2.3%;

12. Mexico - 1.9%;

•   Other countries - 33.9%

I was surprised by these results, because when we think of security issues on the Internet, and hackers, most security experts think of highly trained people working mainly in Eastern Europe – but spam is different from hacking. Spam is primarily a commercial marketing phenomenon, and that explains why such a high proportion comes from within the USA.

So what can you do about it? Firstly most good Internet Service Providers have filters which they set to cut out well known, or notorious, spammers. There are some other simple options that you can use to minimize the amount of junk email that comes in, and to deal with it when it arrives. I strongly suggest you think several times before sending messages to news groups or give personal details to a website, subscribe cautiously to discussion groups and certainly use your email program's filtering system. Some people use several email addresses, keeping separate addresses for personal and business matters.

But what to do when the junk email starts arriving? A colleague of mine, who had been a member of an anti-cult discussion group, suddenly started getting hundreds of messages per day from cults all over the world. They had obtained his address and were determined to stop his right to privacy and free speech. Several other friends have become so desperate they have changed their email address and started all over again – most inconvenient. My personal solution is to read the name of the person who is sending the message and the message title. If neither rings any bells, I simply delete the message unread! If it was a genuine message I know that the sender will phone me or try again. This keeps you sane, and means you cannot possibly be tempted to send large amounts of money to Nigeria, or buy unwanted Viagra!

I advise you to go carefully. There are many Internet sites recommended throughout this book. Visit the sites that interest you. You will learn lots. Go for it sensibly - and good luck!

Key points in this chapter include:

- We are in the time of "Information Age Healthcare"

- There are four key components in effectively searching the web, professional journals/sites, evaluated gateways, generic searches and discussion groups.

- Online technologies are likely to have their greatest effects in preventing illness and in making healthcare more consumer focused

- Virtual Reality environments are rapidly becoming available and offer great promise

6

How To Choose A Doctor On The Net

Ideally your Internet doctor will be the same doctor you see face to face, so you will know each other in both environments, and make a choice as to whether you have your consultations live or in cyberspace, at home or in the surgery, or even by the pool. This is without doubt the best option for you, if you and your doctor wish to work that way. But what if you want to have an Internet doctor, and your usual doctor either is not available like that, or for whatever reason, you prefer to communicate primarily online.

Doctors and therapists on the Internet vary from the very bad to the excellent… with many in between! So how do you choose a good one? I can already see you throwing up your hands in horror …but read on - you *can* sort out a doctor who is right for you! It will take a bit of research but it's better than taking short-cuts and maybe ending up with the wrong person.

Dr Tom Ferguson, who tragically died aged 62 in 2006, was one of the giants of the early years of the Internet. He urged patients to educate themselves and share knowledge with one another, and encouraged doctors to collaborate with patients rather than command them. Predicting the Internet's potential for disseminating medical information long before it became a familiar conduit, he was an early proponent of its use, terming laymen who did so "e-patients." In his influential reports at <u>www.fergusonreport.</u><u>com</u> , which are still archived, he classified doctor's consultation styles on the net into two types. He talked about Type 1 doctors who are "advisors, coaches and information providers" but who specifically do not attempt to diagnose or treat. These doctors, or other health professionals, are typically available through their own sites, or through the many commercial sites. They generally don't advise the same patient twice, usually don't even give their name, although the commercial sites "guarantee" that they are fully qualified, and will often refer you to a local face to face doctor or hospital. Interestingly this is how many of them receive payment for their services - the sites get a "spotters fee" from local services that they refer to - so there is an immediate conflict of interest and potential pressure on the type 1 doctors to refer only to particular local health providers who have agreed to pay this fee.!.

I am deliberately not recommending any particular doctors from these sites because it is really impossible to tell how good they are, although there are many such sites easily accessible via Google. Interestingly a recent study undertaken by ABC's "Good Morning America" found that, while consultations from three major web sites could be useful for routine problems, the sites doctors might make misleading diagnoses in more difficult cases. The program concluded that patients should avoid online consults for problems that couldn't wait more than 24 hours, but that it would be reasonable to consult with their regular physician online about routine problems that they had had before.

Ferguson's type 2 doctors are the majority of medical providers on the net. These are doctors like me who provide normal face to face care, and who encourage their patients to also use email to contact them directly - a rational and sensible use of new technologies which, as long as the guidelines for Internet consultations discussed in this book, are followed, is a great way of working for both patient and doctor. There is another group of health care providers, however, who attempt to provide full health services only on the Internet. Many of these provide counseling or therapy services for mental health problems, or alternative therapies of an often bizarre and inappropriate nature. At the present time my advice is generally to stay away from many of these, unless you can be sure who they are, and ideally can also see them face to face. Full time Internet health services and providers will become much more common in the next few years, however, as we move to being able to use secure video systems over the Internet, and I predict that as many as 10-20% of all health consultations will take place in cyberspace within 10 years or so. This will be a real revolution in healthcare.

Nowadays it's quite usual for patients to "check out" doctors and other health professionals before they visit them but, until recently it was hard to find out much mainly because of advertising restrictions. Patients had to depend on second hand information and opinions. But times have changed. Several patients have come to me after reading my curriculum vitae on the UC Davis website at www.ucdmc.ucdavis.edu/psychiatry, or through having heard of me through a search engine. They chose me for my particular areas of expertise and skills, and made appointments directly with me rather than relying only on their family doctor's choice, or on the advice of neighbor or friend.

Unfortunately, though, most people still fall upon their doctors by chance. Maybe you get a name from a friend, a neighbor or just a chance acquaintance at the corner store. Maybe your doctor or health professional refers you, or an advertisement catches your eye. Sometimes you've no choice and you're referred through the health system because there are only so many providers that are allowable by your insurance group. In future you'll always be able to check out the credentials of your potential caregiver on the Internet, or even find a good doctor from scratch there. Unfortunately many doctors are still not well profiled online, even now in 2008. You can however go to the Medical Board of California and see the profile of every registered doctor in the state, including me, to make sure that they have no license restrictions, or disciplinary actions against them. And this applies whether you intend to see your doctor online, or face to face, whether they have a particular specialty, or live close by you.

INTERNET THERAPY - A GROWTH INDUSTRY.

Therapy is big business in the health world, and becoming very popular on the Internet. Most family doctors spend about a third or more of their time helping people with stress related problems, never mind the number of counselors, psychologists and psychiatrists who see individuals for therapy as well. Using the Internet for counseling or psychotherapy is still in its infancy but it's expanding rapidly. Nobody knows just how many therapists work online. One of the problems is that therapy goes under so many names: counseling, web-therapy, cybertherapy, online therapy, e-therapy, individualized information, individualized advice, behavioral telehealth, Internet health provision and Internet interactions to name a few! When I recently put the word "counselor" into the Google search engine it returned over 30 million mentions on websites, while the word "therapist" returned over 40 million pages! If you put "Internet therapy" into Google you will find over 3 million returned sites, but more interestingly there are 20 sponsored sites – counseling services that have paid Google to display their links. It is impossible to tell how many therapists, and of what quality, work through these 20 paid sites alone, but it is likely in the hundreds at least.

Let's look first at practitioners who say they are specifically interested in mental health, and who provide paid services on the Internet. One of the first studies was undertaken in 1998 when Terri Powell from the University of Kentucky sent out a questionnaire to the fifty online practitioners listed with the Metanoia.com website. This is still one of the most comprehensive listings of mental health practitioners. While only 13 of the counselors replied, back in 1997 they "saw" a total of 1344 clients an average of three times each. The year before 8 therapists worked with 947 clients and the year before that 7 therapists worked with just 445 clients. In other words, this small group of practitioners doubled in size and tripled its number of clients in only 2 years in the early years of the Internet! The site itself includes an interesting historical review of the development of e-therapy up until 2002. Nowadays a substantial number of counselors work through the website – it is worth looking at how the site describes the effectiveness of online therapy:

"Is e-therapy effective?

Meeting face-to-face is still better, but e-therapy can be effective, especially if psychotherapy is not accessible to you.

Working with a therapist online will never replace traditional, face-to-face therapy relationships. No one is suggesting that e-therapy is "better". But that's not the point. E-therapy is not meant to replace traditional therapy; it is another way of caring, one that can reach people who are not getting any other help.

Does e-therapy help people? Yes. Over 90% of the people who work with a therapist online say that it helped them.

Many people cannot, or will not, go to a therapist's office. For them, psychotherapy is not accessible. What keeps people from getting help?

- A person may be too embarrassed, or too uncomfortable to make an appointment with a therapist.

- A person may live in a remote area, far from any therapist's office.

- Scheduling, money, physical challenge, conflicting relationships, or misconceptions keep people from seeking help.

If this describes you, e-therapy may be a place to start"

A TYPICAL NET THERAPIST

In her study Powell painted an interesting picture of what she called the composite Internet counselor. Having reviewed a number of recent websites I suspect her description is still fairly accurate:

"A 48 year old male psychologist with 15 years experience in traditional clinical practice. He's been in online practice for almost 2 years and calls his service, 'advice giving'. When you visit his website, you'll find that he uses some sort of encryption software to protect your anonymity. In order to reduce fraud and exploitation, his credentials have been authenticated. He believes that online mental health services increase clients' access to mental health professionals, especially clients living in remote areas or suffering from disabilities. The average client wants help with relationship problems or depression."

Now let's look at other areas of health and see what Internet doctors are available for general medical problems. You can have almost any question you want answered by a type 1 doctor on the Internet, usually within a few minutes, but with little idea of how experienced the doctor is who is answering you, and little recourse if the information is wrong. There is no overall reliable listing of doctors on the Internet, but they are not difficult to find. Use the search strategy described earlier. Remember that the large commercial sites receive literally millions of hits per month so they are unlikely to be able to provide personal service. If you want more than type 1 consults however, particularly if you wish to receive the majority of your treatment via the Internet, all I can suggest is that you search by your illness or need, in a structured way, and then ask the questions in this chapter.

Do I Want an Online Doctor?

Ideally you will have a doctor you can trust who you can choose to see face to face, or online, depending on your choice and mutual convenience. But there are many situations where you will need to choose a specific doctor who you will consult online, and this will become increasingly common in future as health becomes a global industry. After all why shouldn't you consult a doctor in Australia who is acknowledged as a world expert in say, liver disease, if your usual doctor in New York is uncertain as to your best treatment regime? Even more so if the Australian doctor is cheaper on the Internet than your own because of the weakness of the Australian dollar in comparison to the US dollar!

Look back through the descriptions of people who might benefit from eHealthcare. Do you fall into any of the categories? Maybe you simply prefer eHealthcare to face-to-face.

Check out your options...speak to your doctor, go to the library, discuss your situation with your family, friends or partner and, if you are already seeing a doctor face-to-face, with them as well. You may decide to see an online doctor face-to–face for one session for a comprehensive diagnostic assessment, which should be conducted in a manner similar to that described in Chapter 4, before continuing to see them on the Internet afterwards. Alternatively you may simply decide to do some surfing and access health information about your condition - use the approaches recommended in this book in chapter 5 and the sites suggested in the appendix.

If, by now, you believe eHealth is right for you then it is time to look for an online doctor or health professional. You may have already found one in the course of your investigations but I still strongly suggest that you follow the guidelines in this chapter. Ask your doctor or therapist the questions in the second half of this chapter and be wary if they cannot, or will not, answer them. And don't forget to assess their website as well in accord with the suggestions later in this chapter, perhaps using the tool available at the Discern website.(www.discern.org.uk).

FACE TO FACE, OR ONLINE?

If you are already seeing a face to face doctor but would like to consult an online health professional as well, then explain this to your doctor who needs to know so that mixed therapeutic messages do not occur that may not be in your best interest. Your usual doctor may also be able to give you the extra help you want. Don't give up on your face to face doctor too quickly. EHealthcare is still relatively new. We know it can be effective, that it's an important adjunct to other treatment approaches but until it's clearer in which areas it's most effective, it shouldn't be automatically assumed to be better than face to face care. In fact it's probably not in many instances.

Now let's look at some individual health professional's sites. Many of them are offering counseling. To give you a feel for what's on offer I have selected excerpts from individual web pages. All these sites profess to employ professionally qualified clinicians with either medical, masters or PhD degrees. Some sound good and some not so good! You'll recognize why as we explore what to look out for later in this chapter.

"Whether you need general guidance, are on the verge of a crisis, or are looking for competent peer review YYY may be able to help. We are not a substitute for face to face therapy, and may not be appropriate for everyone, but we do focus the attention of a group of highly skilled professionals on YOU! These are the same people who normally charge $100 to $200 per session!□□ *You need not send us your name, address or even phone number if you do not wish*□□*. All charges are discreetly billed to your credit card, and the therapist never sees your billing information."*

"XXX is the only Internet site that provides a LIVE physician-based interaction for patients in the comfort of their own home – a virtual house call!! Whether at home, at school, or traveling within the country or abroad, XXX provides real-time, online, confidential consultative medical advice for our patients on the Internet"

"My professional counseling rate is kept low, so you can afford it: just $90 per hour, charged to your credit card□□..If you want to remain anonymous, it is not necessary to tell me your real name, even though you use a credit card. I understand that the issues you need to deal with may be nearly impossible for you to be open about under your actual name. So if you prefer, give me an alternate "working" name□□.I genuinely look forward to hearing from you□to getting to know you and understand youv □.to gently exploring your areas of difficulty and pain□.to achieving what none of us can do alone."

"Welcome to the first 24 hour telephone and online counseling service. There is no subject that is taboo. Whether your situation deals with sex, a relationship, gender issues, a past or present trauma in your life, substance abuse or addictions, eating disorders, a problem at work or home, depression, anxiety, phobias, parenting, an illness or just about anything else, we are here for you. All our counselors are licensed professionals (with Masters or PhD degrees) who care deeply about their clients and who work very hard to help them achieve the good health and peace of mind they desire in their lives. That's our goal."

Whichever treatment or online assessment and consultation you are considering you should get a description of the philosophy behind the practitioner's approach, what type of consultation you are being offered and how long it will take. Ask these questions at the very beginning.

Obviously the doctor will have to perform a detailed assessment of your situation before being able to answer such questions. This assessment, in most clinical situations, normally takes at least an hour and may involve you filling in questionnaires and/or taking some tests. If you do not receive such an assessment, either by email, phone, face to face or even by videoconference, forget that health professional! How can they possibly know how to help you if they haven't taken the trouble to find out about you?

People choose their doctors with several factors in mind. Many people choose by gender - females, in particular, often prefer to see a female doctor. We also look at the therapist's expertise or experience with our problem. But, most commonly, we choose by price or availability - not a great way to guarantee a successful doctor/patient relationship! You wouldn't choose a car without checking it out…nor should you choose a doctor that way. Particularly when you are on the modern day equivalent of the Wild West - the world wide web.

Assessing Your E-Doctor - Ten Questions to Ask

You know now how *not* to choose a doctor, but how *do* you find the right one? There are ten questions you should ask. We'll look at each of the questions then work through how a good online doctor should respond. Remember to be friendly, businesslike, and don't take "no" for an answer. You are paying for the consultation. You are the customer. You must be satisfied with both the consultation and the consultant. These rules apply equally for an online or face to face health professional.
Ask:

- What are your qualifications and credentials?

- What experience do you have in offering face-to-face and e-care?

- Are you registered to practice in your own state or country, and mine, (if you are in a different country) and do you have appropriate malpractice insurance?

- Do you adhere to a documented code of ethics? Which one?

- What clinical and administrative guidelines for practice do you use?

- What areas do you have expertise in, and what evidence in the form of professional recognition, publications or lectures do you have to confirm this?

- Do you communicate with colleagues for continuing medical education, professional supervision and self-development?

- Do you provide face to face support for your online patients if required?

- What are your billing procedures?

- Do you record consultations electronically in any way and, if so, what are your consent and confidentiality procedures for this. How do you keep your clinical records, both face-to-face and online?

What are your qualifications and credentials?

No doctor or ethical health professional from any background should mind being asked about their qualifications. They should be proud of their achievements. Indeed many doctors in office practice hang their qualification certificates in their rooms so patients can examine them. Generally you should ensure your e-consultant has a medical degree or masters/doctoral level qualification in another relevant health profession. Many websites, and most large institutions, proudly include detailed biographies of the doctors who practice through them and you should always check these details before consulting with any doctor on the web or face to face. I am personally very wary of sites, and there are many, who simply say that they offer consultations by qualified doctors but who do not give out the names and details of these physicians. Would you go and consult a doctor in the face to face world if you did not even know their name, never mind what their qualifications were?

The bottom line is that doctors offering e-care should have their credentials on a website. At the very least the site should contain details of their professional degrees and qualifications. It should also have a Curriculum Vitae showing academic and professional training, courses attended, special interests and expertise and any research papers or scientific publications they've contributed to. If they advertise a particular expertise there should be evidence to support this such as higher training or teaching and research skills. Doctors should always be prepared to answer questions about their credentials and their contact details should be found on the webpage. It's also great to find their photo. Photos contain lots of extra, often subconscious, information. The website may also contain links to the relevant pages of their professional organization where you should find relevant ethical guidelines.

I believe it won't be too long before professional associations develop licensing for online practitioners. This will mean, for example, that the American Psychiatric Association will be able to tell you which psychiatrists meet the ethical and clinical requirements that the Association develops for e-therapies. The same will be true for the British Medical Association and other professional bodies for both specialist and generalist practitioners. It will make the search for reputable e-practitioners much easier.

It is obviously not easy for patients to decide whether someone with a Masters degree in Education is an expert in asthma advice and management or whether a PhD in research methods equips a person to practice online hypnotherapy! Health practitioners come from many different backgrounds and unfortunately in many cases their training is non-existent or, perhaps worse, biased by their own philosophies or perspectives on life. Or they may simply be frauds.

My advice is if an online health practitioner from any discipline is not registered with a professional organization, don't go near them! Ask for their registration number so you can independently contact that professional body to confirm their membership. And do that.

No *Nom de Plumes*!

It worries me that many of the e-practitioners on the net offer health services without needing to know your real name and address. This is amazingly unprofessional. Doctors who belong to professional associations are obliged to offer help to patients in crisis situations. How can you do this if you don't know who your clients really are?

I believe that if someone is happy to give you consultations online without insisting on knowing who you are and where you live, then you should definitely move on to someone else. Such "practitioners" are usually more interested in your credit card than you. Of course, anonymous one-off advice sessions through such well recognized organizations as Samaritans and Lifeline are fine but otherwise offering consultations anonymously is simply bizarre. If the online doctor won't tell you their name and license number go elsewhere - it is not good enough for the site to boast, as several do, that "all our doctors are board certified" if the individual doctor you are consulting, or who is answering your questions, won't say who they are. Why should you pay for a service when you don't know who is providing it?

What experience do you have in face-to-face healthcare?

An online practitioner should already be an experienced face to face professional. Online consultations are more demanding than face to face ones; there are more potential pitfalls and greater organizational and ethical traps for the unwary. Except in exceptional circumstances I don't believe anyone should offer online consultations without at least five years full time face to face health experience. Don't be sucked into seeing someone who is clinically inexperienced. Ask them about it. If they can't prove their experience, move on. It doesn't happen yet, but in future online doctors may even have to provide testimonies of their skills from previously treated patients, just as happens when you choose a builder or architect. Why should doctors be so different from other professions?

Most online clinicians of the future will have secure websites where they will describe their skills and experience, communicate with patients and market their services. To check the quality of their site and the experience of the doctor, go through the following checklist:

1. Who is the author of the site?Perform a Medline or Psycinfo search as detailed later in this chapter to check out both the site author and the doctor.Frequently they are the same person.

2. Which institution supports the doctor and what affiliations do they have?Do they have an MD from Harvard as opposed to a diploma from the Dreamtime University of Angola?

3. Are the author and the doctor identified and can they be contacted?Avoid all health websites that don't have some sort of feedback or quality control mechanism. And give them your feedback whether you like them, and the site, or not.

4. Is the information on the website current?Check out (usually at the bottom of the homepage) when the site was last updated and how often this occurs.

5. Is the information on the website balanced?I have yet to find a health care issue with only one side to an argument or piece of advice.Even if the evidence for one particular approach is overwhelming, there will always be people who disagree and they should be represented, or at least mentioned.Reputable sites will discuss possible biases, and will also declare any possible interests, particularly sponsorship related conflicts of interest.

6. Can you verify the information on the website - particularly via hotlinks to other unrelated sites which are managed by different groups of people or organizations?Links to public libraries, universities and government agencies suggest better quality information than links to commercial organizations, unusual religious sects or political parties!

Most importantly, find out if the website is trying to sell you something? Many health sites are linked to expensive "natural products" and the site is really no more than a shop front for them. You should be skeptical about websites which have significant commercial sponsorship or advertising.

In general look for sites displaying the logo saying that the site is set up according to the principles of the Health on the Net Foundation (HON) (www.hon.ch/HON/Conduct.html). This is a not-for-profit organization founded in 1995 under the auspices of the Geneva Ministry of Health and based in Switzerland. The HON came about following the gathering of 36 experts to discuss the growing concerns over the unequal quality of online health information. The mission of the foundation is to help both laypersons and medical practitioners find useful and reliable medical and health information online.

The HON Code is not designed to rate the veracity of the information provided by a Web site. The code only states that the site holds to the standards, so that you can know the source and purpose of the medical information presented. It is the oldest and the most used ethical and trustworthy code for medical and health related information available on the Internet and is currently used by over 5000 certified websites, covering 72 countries and 34 languages.

The principles of the HONcode are:

1. Authority - information and advice given only by medical professionals with credentials of author/s, or a clear statement if this is not the case

2. Complementarity - information and help are to support, not replace, patient-healthcare professional relationships which is the desired means of contact

3. Confidentiality - how the site treats personal and non-personal information of readers

4. Attribution - references to source of information (URL if available online)and dates when pages was last updated

5. Justifiability - any treatment, product or service must be supported by balanced, well-referenced scientific information

6. Transparency of authorship - contact information, preferably including email addresses, of authors should be available

7. Transparency of sponsorship - sources of funding for the site

8. Honesty in advertising and editorial policy - details about advertising on the site and clear distinction between advertised and editorial material

At www.mentalhealth.com Dr Phillip Long, the psychiatrist editor of Internet Mental Health, shows how to spot websites which depend heavily on corporate sponsorship. In one of his examples a sponsor's pharmaceutical product is mentioned 31 times with no references to any rival medications! He describes many hidden links between the pharmaceutical industry and medical education programs, both face to face, and online. Examples include The Washington Post exposure of the hidden link between a major health insurer, Aetna, and a very popular health portal which advertised itself as "The Trusted Source". Odd how such a trusted source couldn't tell consumers who owned it! Hence you won't find me recommending commercial health portals in this book that do not at least support the principles of the Health on the Net Foundation.

In reality sponsorship of websites is probably here to stay and it's likely that some popular sites will be heavily sponsored by unrelated products.

Search engines, computer companies and www.Amazon.com, the huge online bookstore, already advertise on many health sites and, as long as there is no unhealthy conflict of interest, this should be encouraged. Just remember that the advertisements are there to sell products, while you are there to find information – very different motivating factors.

Disclaimers are found on most health websites. Many online practitioners state they are providing information, not giving proper health services, and are not to blame if the information is wrong or irrelevant. A fairly typical disclaimer on a site offering health information, discussion groups and chat lists, but not attempting to provide online consultations, reads like this:

"The diagnosis and treatment of disease requires trained medical professionals. The information provided below is to be used for educational purposes only. It should NOT be used as a substitute for seeking professional care."

Does your normal face to face treatment work - are you an effective doctor either face to face or on the net?

Last but by no means least, don't forget to ask your potential e-doctor how many patients with your particular problem they have treated. How did those patients respond to the treatment and if you are one of the unlucky ones who don't recover in the expected manner, what would they do?! The answer to these questions is crucial. Many major hospitals now post health outcome parameters on their websites, and some states literally run "league tables" comparing, for instance, survival outcomes from different cardiac surgery programs. Check with your doctor what outcome measures, if any, have been used to measure their practice, and who they are compared against. And ask to see the results. If you are not happy with the answer, move on to the next doctor, or perhaps check in with the program that has the best survival figures.

Are you registered to practice in your state or country and mine? Do you have malpractice insurance?

All reputable online practitioners will be registered with a health licensing board, professional indemnity insurance company or professional association. Most will be with all three. You should arm yourself your doctor's registration number and contact the associations to confirm they are legally registered to practice. In the United States many registration bodies only allow doctors to practice in one state however elsewhere it is more common for them to be registered to practice throughout their country. Make sure your practitioner is registered to practice not only in their state but in your state as well if you are being treated across state boundaries. International registration is cowboy country and at this stage international medical licenses valid in multiple countries simply do not exist! The closest qualification to a global license is the US Medical Licensing Examination (USMLE) because the same number of non-US trained doctors, as US trainees, take it every year. In the future global medical registration is inevitable but currently all that doctors can do is register in all countries where they practice. This can be extremely difficult because of the different registration systems, standards and laws.

In some parts of the USA the potential legal ramifications of e-care malpractice are causing considerable disquiet. Luckily this doesn't appear to be such a problem in other countries where suing one's doctor isn't such a popular pastime. For patients, though, the bottom line is to make sure that your doctor is fully licensed and carries appropriate malpractice insurance cover. Otherwise you have no comeback if things go wrong.

What code of ethics do you work by?

It is vital, and essential, that your online health practitioner adheres to a code of ethics - a set of rules and principles that govern the way they practice. Assuming they belong to a professional body they will use that body's code of ethics which you should be able to read on their web page. For example have a look at the website for the American Medical Association (www.ama-assn.org) where the AMA code of ethics is prominently posted, and reads as follows:

"The medical profession has long subscribed to a body of ethical statements developed primarily for the benefit of the patient. As a member of this profession, a physician must recognize responsibility to patients first and foremost, as well as to society, to other health professionals, and to self. The following Principles adopted by the American Medical Association are not laws, but standards of conduct which define the essentials of honorable behavior for the physician.

Principles of medical ethics

I.   A physician shall be dedicated to providing competent medical care, with compassion and respect for human dignity and rights.

II. A physician shall uphold the standards of professionalism, be honest in all professional interactions, and strive to report physicians deficient in character or competence, or engaging in fraud or deception, to appropriate entities.

III. A physician shall respect the law and also recognize a responsibility to seek changes in those requirements which are contrary to the best interests of the patient.

IV. A physician shall respect the rights of patients, colleagues, and other health professionals, and shall safeguard patient confidences and privacy within the constraints of the law.

V.   A physician shall continue to study, apply, and advance scientific knowledge, maintain a commitment to medical education, make relevant information available to patients, colleagues, and the public, obtain consultation, and use the talents of other health professionals when indicated.

VI.   A physician shall, in the provision of appropriate patient care, except in emergencies, be free to choose whom to serve, with whom to associate, and the environment in which to provide medical care.

VII.   A physician shall recognize a responsibility to participate in activities contributing to the improvement of the community and the betterment of public health.

VIII.   A physician shall, while caring for a patient, regard responsibility to the patient as paramount.

IX.   A physician shall support access to medical care for all people."

Because it is vital that practitioners have the highest ethical principles and standards you should always choose a person who has a specific professional background and training and who uses a set of ethical rules and guidelines to guide their professional practice. There are many cowboys on the Internet who don't operate under these ethics and if you use them you are at their mercy!

What clinical and administrative guidelines do you use?

Most reputable online practitioners adapt treatment and administrative guidelines published by professional bodies to suit their own personal style, philosophy and skills. Check that yours does. Guidelines are available in many areas of healthcare, for individual types of practice, for differing situations, and especially for particular disorders or interventions. The terms "best practice" and "evidence based" are typically used in association with guidelines, and usually indicate that there has been a reasonably comprehensive quality assurance process or methodology used by the writers of the guidelines. One essential stop for any patient should be the National Guideline clearinghouse (NGC) at www.guideline.gov. Here you can find almost any guideline on any subject in a comprehensive database of evidence-based clinical practice guidelines and related documents. The NGC is an initiative of the Agency for Healthcare Research and Quality (AHRQ), and the U.S. Department of Health and Human Services and was originally created in partnership with the American Medical Association and the American Association of Health Plans

The following are some examples of a variety of guidelines relevant to eHealth:

GUIDELINES FOR EMAIL

The American Informatics Association (www.amia.org) has published guidelines for doctors using email for clinical and administrative purposes. Among their recommendations are:

- Don't use e-mail for urgent matters, use the phone or personal communications as you can't be sure when email will be answered.

- Ensure that patients know who reads your email, how and where the emails are stored and whether copies are made and placed in your health care notes.

- Decide with patients what type of transactions they should undertake using email, and define the type of transaction in the subject line of the message so you can filter it quickly when reading your email. Where possible use codes known only to you and the patient.

- Ensure patients know they should phone you or your consulting rooms if they don't get a response within an agreed period of time, say 48 hours.

- Agree not to forward possibly identifiable material about the patient to a third party without their express consent.

- Use encrypted email, if possible. This isn't always possible because encryption has to occur at both ends. If it is not practicable ensure that the patient understands that the email is not secure.

TELE-HOME CARE GUIDELINES

Guidelines for patients receiving homecare through telemedicine, videoconferencing using broad bandwidth, can be found on the American Telemedicine Association's website at http://atmeda.org., as can guidelines for the practice of ophthalmology online. These guidelines are indicative of the sort of guidelines that will have to be introduced to eHealthcare on the net once video consultations are easily available over the Internet and real time video consultations with your doctor become more common, especially from the home. Some of the more important points in the homecare guidelines are:

For Patients: "The first and last visit to the patient's home must be in person and not by video visit; patients may un-enroll from tele-homecare at any time; patients (or their caregivers) must be able to use and maintain the equipment and patients may not be viewed through the video without their knowledge or prior written consent."

For the provider: " Personnel providing tele-home care must document each video visit in the patient's chart; they may only make video visits within the limits of their expertise, a physician order must be obtained to integrate tele-home care into the care plan, and, if 24 hour tele-home care is not available, patients must be provided with written instructions for contacting after-hours care providers."

What are your areas of expertise? What evidence do you have in the form of professional recognition, publications or lectures?

Some health practitioners boast expertise in the most weird and wonderful things! Expertise in Projective Dynamism or Compulsive Dissociation sounds very important…but they are not recognized specialties! In fact I have just made both of these up, so beware!

Good doctors also teach; many carry out research. Increasingly doctors will have their qualifications, research references and teaching expertise detailed on their home pages but that is still relatively uncommon at present. There are other ways to check up however - all you need to do is perform a literature or Internet search.

Do you have access to colleagues for continuing medical education (CME), and for professional supervision and self-development? Do you provide face to face support for your online patients if required?

Isolated doctors are potentially dangerous. Most doctors have close ties with colleagues with whom they can discuss their most difficult patients for support and advice. Good practitioners realize they don't know everything and are always seeking external reviews of their practice and opportunities to extend their learning. All licensed US doctors have to undertake mandated numbers of hours of accredited continuing medical education – usually between 25-100 hours per year, depending on the State licensing authorities. A potential downside of online healthcare is that doctors who spend much of their time online may not get the interaction with colleagues which is so important, but at the same time large numbers of CME programs are now offered online, with sites such as WebMD/Medscape undertaking 17% of all CME accredited hours nationally.

Your e-doctor must have a back up system in place so patients who are in severe crisis or are acutely unwell can receive immediate treatment and assistance in their own environment at any time. This is because most doctors only log on at certain times of the day and patients may have to wait 24 hours for a response to an email. This is obviously dangerously inadequate in emergency situations.

Legitimate email therapists working through reasonable sites such as www.metanoia.org in the area of mental health, advise their patients what to do in an emergency:

"If you are having suicidal thoughts you may need help immediately. Take yourself seriously. If your need is urgent, admit it. You deserve to get help, and to get it sooner rather than later. If you are experiencing intense emotional distress and need immediate response

Get off the computer and pick up the phone.

Telephone a mental health hotline (numbers in your phone book)

Otherwise call a psychotherapist, counseling centre or mental health clinic and make an appointment for an office visit. In urgent situations many therapists will see you on short notice. Be sure to make it clear that your need is urgent."

Suicidal persons might wish to read this first".

This last message is in hypertext and links to some excellent advice from an anonymous patient aimed at persuading suicidal people to reconsider.

How Do You Bill?

Billing for online services has to be transparent and agreed to in advance of any consultations. Frauds abound on the Internet …sadly common are the charlatans who set up non-secure websites then charge $20 to $50 per question on any health subject! You have no guarantee the answer will be individual to you, has come from a particular therapist or is even correct! I have even found sites that won't give you any information about the site or the therapist unless you pay the question fee up front! The only thing you can guarantee is they're happy to take your credit card through the only secure part of the site!

You are better to pay a well qualified doctor by the hour to answer your questions, rather than pay by the question. Hourly costs vary from about $30 to $100. Not only will you get much better value, your chance of getting the same practitioner for follow-up questions is much greater.

When paying for health services with a credit card NEVER put your credit card number in ordinary email and NEVER use an unsecured website. Insist on using either traditional mail or bank transfer, a secure Internet payment service such as paypal or a site accredited by VeriSign (your browser should tell you if it's secure) or fax or telephone your credit care number through to the doctor - making sure that the number you are ringing really does belong to the doctor. If your online practitioner rejects these options assume it's a scam and don't pay.

Do you record any sessions electronically? If so what are your consent and confidentiality procedures for this and for your records of sessions both face-to-face and online?

Confidentiality is crucial for any doctor, and even more so for the online practitioner. Fixed telephone lines are more secure than mobile phones. Remember Prince Charles and his embarrassing intimate conversations with his then mistress Camilla Parker-Bowles! Ideally email messages should be encrypted although this doesn't always happen. At the very least your doctor should check with you to ensure you received their email, and should adhere to the email guidelines given earlier in this chapter. After all emails do disappear into Cyberspace, never to be seen again!

You must find out how your doctor keeps his or her clinical notes. How safe are these? Who else can access them? Most doctors using email simply print out and file their clinical emails into paper based records at present. This is a far more accurate record than note-taking during a verbal exchange.

If you are not sure that your email messages are confidential, forget it. The following scenarios could make you think twice!

An employee receiving email counseling at his work address finds his email is being read (legally) by his boss. The embarrassed employee is fired and ends up more distressed than ever.

An explicit email from a patient to his doctor is accidentally sent to an entire email list of several thousand people resulting in excruciatingly public humiliation.

A wife reads her husband's email in which he admits infidelity with other women and declares his love for his online doctor. She emails them both to acquaint them of her discovery, sends a copy of her husband's email to her lawyer, changes the locks on the house and plots urgent re-constructive surgery on his genitals.

By choosing the right online doctor you shouldn't end up in situations like these! Don't rush your choice, ask him or her the questions in this chapter and if you are satisfied with the answers you should be reasonably confident that you have found a professional eHealthcare practitioner. But don't forget that the best online doctor, is also your face to face doctor.

WRAPPING IT UP - BRINGING IT ALL TOGETHER

In short, the effective online doctor of the future will be:

- an experienced face to face doctor - competent and consumer focused;

- able to understand, integrate and use a variety of information technologies - also know when not to use them;

- respectful of his patients and able to work with them in a partnership;

- trained in individual and group communication techniques;

- an expert communicator with good media skills;

- able to evaluate and analyze large amounts of health information, prioritize and provide best practice treatments;

- constantly updating himself and evaluating his own practice and the therapeutic outcomes of his patients.

Find yourself someone who embodies all these ideals and you have found yourself the perfect online doctor!

7

Changing Relationships

It doesn't seem very long ago (actually it was 1979!) that as a raw young medical student I made my first rounds in an antiquated London hospital which, thankfully, no longer exists. The patients, terrified into submission by a ferocious senior nurse were laid out for the pleasure of the parading surgeon and his cortege of nurses and students. These patients were not allowed to speak as the surgeon made pronouncements and decisions of great import, all the while tapping them patronizingly on the heads! The only expectation of the patients was that they look suitably grateful. If a patient had the audacity to question a decision they were likely to labeled as noncompliant, a troublemaker or having an "inadequate personality". I remember another student telling me the only way to tell whether a patient on that ward was bleeding internally was to lift up the blankets at the bottom of the bed and see if the sheets were red! Thank heavens things have changed!

Today, patient - doctor relationships are much better. Online systems have exposed patients to a huge amount of health information helping them to have an informed say in their own health care. This is balancing the scales of the patient -doctor relationship - medical paternalism will soon be consigned to the history books forever. This is probably the most significant way that the Internet can improve your healthcare – it gives you the power of information and levels the playing field between you and your doctor. And it does this in a very positive way, that not only aids your health, but which has advantages for both you and your doctor – a real win-win situation.

THE TWO FACES OF YOUR DOCTOR – THE THERAPEUTIC RELATIONSHIP

There are two components to the doctor-patient relationship: the empathetic component - how well the doctor understands you, how he thinks and makes decisions to tailor numerous possible treatment options to you as an individual; and the technical component - the expert knowledge which your doctor has learnt and uses for your betterment.

Professor Richard Wootton, who currently directs the Scottish Telemedicine network, believes that many people regard an excellent doctor-patient relationship as the gold standard in health care delivery. Sadly many patients today are dissatisfied with the traditional 'doctors know best' attitude and Wootton believes that the emphasis on good communication in online relationships may mean that doctor-patient rapport will improve and regain its former high status. Clearly patients expect consultations to encompass both art and science. If you are interested in the way doctors make decisions, and how they think, I encourage you to read the best selling book by Jerome Groopman, MD, called "How Doctors Think". It is a fascinating paradox that a side effect of our technologically sophisticated age is the resurgence of good language and written skills as we see happening on the Internet.

DOCTOR-PATIENT RELATIONSHIPS

In traditional face-to-face care there are two typical therapeutic relationship styles – the active - dependent relationship and the mutual participation, or partnership, relationship. With the evolution of online therapy two new levels of relationship will evolve – the pre-therapy stage of self and family care, and the patient driven relationship, where the doctor is merely an adviser, albeit an expert one. Armed with information for the first time in history patients are able to literally "turn off" their doctor with the click of a mouse. This single factor will dramatically alter the power structure of the relationship.

In the traditional **active - dependent relationship** the physician is dominant, possibly even controlling and paternalistic while the patient is mostly dependent and accepting. Patients have some choices but they tend to play the role of passive follower behind an expert leader. This relationship is appropriate in certain online situations especially early in the assessment process or when a clinician is using expert knowledge to advise on and teach about an illness. However, it will become less common in future as patients become increasingly empowered and knowledgeable.

The other relationship is of **mutual participation.** This is the ideal face-to-face relationship for most purposes. It implies equality, trust and collaboration with both participants needing and depending on the other's input. This is the relationship that I try to achieve with my face to face patients in the offline world. Ideally this is the relationship you will have with your doctor, whether you are online or face to face.

Now let's look at online relationships.

INFORMED PATIENTS

As patients become more knowledgeable, or are "information rich," they will increasingly become the main driving force in the doctor-patient relationship.

EHealth heralds a new **pre-therapy relationship** phase where patients research, often with their family and friends, their problem or situation. Access to type 1 consultations will be particularly important here. It will become increasingly easy to discover high quality reliable diagnostic and general information, but at the same time doctors will also be researched, and their skills examined. All doctors of the future will have Internet home pages and patients will increasingly be able to make rational informed decisions about the sort of doctor, and the type of relationship and treatment, that they want. In most cases patients will have carried out the research even before they have consulted the doctor, either face to face, or online. Patients will be able to define who, when, how and where the relationship will occur. Doctors will have to lay out their wares, their skills, their products, to an increasingly savvy group of patients. Surgeons will detail their infection rates, physicians their drug interaction rates, and pediatricians their philosophies for treating children with cancer. Ultimately it should be possible to select a doctor in a similar way to the manner we now use for airline tickets or hotels – on a website, by specialty, availability, price and insurance situation, special skills, outcome measures, geography and so on.

A physician colleague of mine who is an international expert on a very unusual disorder recently told me of his embarrassment when a company executive came to see him about his wife who was said to suffer from this particular disorder. He gave the executive relevant information about the disease, quoted some papers he had written and explained how the man could best help his wife. To his surprise, at the end of the interview, the executive suddenly produced a comprehensive list of 23 case reports of the disease taken from international literature on the Internet. The executive knew more about the recent case reports than did my colleague!

Of course many people will diagnose themselves before even seeing a doctor. I now routinely ask patients what they have read on the Internet, and what they think their diagnosis is. Almost all patients have tried to work out their diagnosis before they see me, and many are right, and have found out about their problem, and validated their symptoms against the numerous questionnaires and diagnostic tools available for almost all disorders. This often makes the assessment I undertake very much easier, and I am therefore able to spend more time than I used to working out the best treatment regime, and educating my patients further. There are a large number of good screening questionnaires on the Internet. To find them just put your presumed diagnosis into Google, along with the term "screening test" or "diagnostic criteria". The beauty of these questionnaires is that you don't need a health professional to be present when you fill them in. Print out your results and discuss them with your doctor as no such diagnostic tests are definitive and it is very important that you have your opinion correctly reviewed and validated. You won't always be right!

The fourth type of relationship is becoming increasingly common. In this relationship the doctor is the adviser, while the **patient drives** the process of the relationship, makes the choices and the decisions, tapping into the doctor's expertise to create their overall treatment plan. The following example comes from my casebook.

I first met John, a 53 year old married plumber, when he was brought into hospital by a squad of police following a siege. John was extremely paranoid and had started shooting at neighbors who he thought were being sent by the devil to kill him. Our initial relationship was an active-dependent one. On my orders John was sedated and placed in seclusion. Over the next few days his psychosis settled with medications but he became overtly depressed and felt extremely guilty about what he had done. As his paranoia decreased our relationship started to become more equal. After leaving hospital he gradually gained in confidence, his mood improved with appropriate therapy and he and his traumatized family began to understand more about his illness.

I had diagnosed John as having a bipolar disorder - manic depression as it used to be known. He became an active member of a consumer support group, collaborating in his treatment and making his own choices as our relationship became one of mutual participation.

A year later he moved with his family to a town several hundred miles away. Although John now receives treatment and monitoring through a primary care physician I still get occasional emails from him. These usually include the latest research findings in bipolar disorder with a request for my comments. For me this move to an online collaborator-commentator relationship is the evolution of a fascinating relationship. John now controls our relationship - quite the opposite of when we first me - and he makes sure I keep up to date with the literature on bipolar disorders!

The patient driven phase of a therapeutic relationship is likely to become increasingly common as patients maintain long term online relationships with their doctors. Patients who are interested in their own illnesses and keep up-to-date with the latest research and clinical findings through libraries and the Internet will feed information to their doctors not only to keep the therapists up-to-date but, more importantly, to obtain the therapists' opinion of the new findings. Many patients will keep their own personal health records online, and will give their doctors access as required. This is just the opposite of what typically happens now of course. And some of these relationships will be prolonged for years because of the ability of both patient and doctor to remain in contact via the Internet even after one of them has moved home, perhaps to a different country. I have one patient from Australia who still contacts me by phone or email every few months even although I have lived in the USA for some years. He usually wants my opinion on any changes to his treatment regime ordered by his Australian doctors, and greatly values my "second opinion."

COMMUNICATING THROUGH OUR SENSES_

One of the greatest human attributes is our ability to communicate - often with style and subtlety. We express ourselves with voice, language, gestures, faces and body language, clothes and makeup, perfumes and hairstyles. We communicate to let others know about ourselves, to attract others and to make statements about how we see ourselves. Communication is the hub of all our relationships. In face to face situations we can see, feel, hear, taste and smell people. Despite a lack of scientific evidence some people believe there is also a "sixth sense" - intuition, more commonly attributed to females than males.

In online relationships several of these senses are altered and we have to either do without them or depend more heavily on other senses. This doesn't have to be a disadvantage. Blind people, for instance, compensate for their loss of vision by increasing their hearing and smell sensitivity and can often pick up environmental or relationship cues from those senses more accurately than sighted people. While the blind cannot see they can still communicate effectively albeit in a different way. This is what happens online.

We use different senses for the various different approaches to eHealth. For example on the telephone we use hearing only, often with a spicing of intuition thrown in. Many people feel less inhibited speaking on the phone and prefer it to communicating face to face. When we communicate using email or the Internet, we use our vision for the written word and other options such as video clips, pictures and drawings. Hearing is becoming increasingly important with Internet telephony and audible email attachments. Email is usually asynchronous communication with interactions occurring sequentially over hours or day, although chat groups and net meetings may be fully interactive.

Posted by Jerrie on bulletin board

I have been with my partner for seven years and have always been faithful – until recently. A colleague at work began flirting with me on email. At first I took no notice but I was flattered and eventually I responded. I won't go into details, but once he gets what he wants he becomes very cold and accusing until, a few days later, the messages begin again. It's the detachedness of the situation, and the secret messages, that turns me on and keeps sending me back to him. I know he is using me, but what I don't understand is why do I repeatedly let him, and why do his messages drive me crazy for him.

Reply by Art.

It seems to me that you are projecting all the qualities you look for in a partner onto your colleague. That is typical of online relationships because you cannot see or hear the other person, so the lack of stimuli and context makes your mind project the qualities you like onto others. Your colleague has proven to you that he is not what you thought he was. Do not jeopardize your solid relationship for a couple of weeks of excitement that will soon go. If you really care about your partner end the online relationship – it's destined to fail sooner or later.

Communication online is obviously different from face to face communication. It will never be as comprehensive or integrated because it's unlikely we'll ever be able to smell or touch each other through a computer, although some researchers are now trying to "code" smells! But it does have some advantages. As our experience of the new technology increases we will be able to communicate more effectively online. This will be a fascinating field for research.

TRANSFERENCE

The possibility of 'transference' in online relationships should be recognized by both patients and doctors. Transference is the transfer of feelings from past events or relationships from the patient to the doctor. Counter-transference is the transfer of the doctor's feelings from past events or relationships to the patient. In the face to face world these feelings can be extremely powerful to the extent that it is not uncommon for patients to fall in love with doctors, (or unfortunately, the reverse), or to act out extreme emotions such as anger, jealousy, rage and anxiety within the relationship. Sensible male doctors ensure that they have a female nurse with them during physical examinations if they are at all worried about this possibility. Unfortunately it is not uncommon for doctors and patients to fall in love - a major ethical sin for a doctor - and this tends to lead to newspaper headlines, court cases and deregistration for the doctor.

In online relationships there is a higher likelihood of transference because the partners may not know as much about each other. This may be because the relationship is happening in only some sensory modalities or because the participants cannot pick up all the usual visual or other sensory cues. There is more uncertainty, more mystery, online. The tendency online is for patients to project more readily onto the doctor, as well as onto others with whom they are having online relationships. This leads to the relatively commonly reported experience where people say that everyone they meet online seems to be similar. They are not similar but are perceived as such because of similar projections onto them. Alternatively the online user may be unconsciously picking up similarities in people that they meet online and self-selecting people for online relationships that fit with their own needs. These transference reactions are further complicated by transference to the computer itself, or to other communications technology which filters the doctor-patient relationship.

Transference and counter transference are also seen in Internet therapy groups as Yvette Colon has described:

"Unlike face to face group therapy, the online group exists only in time and mind. Because the group is available 24 hours per day and provides instant access to members who want to post when they are reflective or mad or inquisitive or thoughtful, response time is not always predictable☐☐ *Because the group members and I did not see each other, it was easy for members to idealize me or project their fantasies and wishes onto me. Because I am unseen and "mysterious", anger and frustration were taken out on me more readily. Conversely my idealization and projection onto clients could be difficult as well. Because I didn't know what the group members looked like, it became easy to accept the personas they created as the group continued."*

OUR E-PERSONA

We all have different personalities and, strange but true, our personalities can change when we are on the computer, especially when we are writing emails. As yet, we don't know much about just how different personality styles are affected by online technology or how different people react and behave in a variety of online situations. The more I use email, the more frequently I find myself not hitting the "send" icon. It is so easy to offend people on email, with no intention, and once an email is sent it cannot be taken back. So if you are an impulsive person who has got into trouble in email conversations you will be someone who gains from what will certainly be plenty of research into the e-persona in the future.

What we can hazard a guess at, though, is how the different personality styles cited in the literature project themselves online. Take the –

Psychopathic/Antisocial personality - Could they be the online hackers and criminals - especially in deception and fraud - of the new millennium? Or are they the online "entrepreneurs" who pop up wherever there's money to be made and ethical principles are loose. Beware online "therapists" who might be in this category.

Narcissistic/Self-loving personality – Perhaps these people are running bulletin boards contributing at inordinate length as the 'experts' and delighting in expelling everyone who disagrees with them. Maybe they're the ones who are heavily into cybersex - there's no chance of their losing face through premature ejaculation or rejection!

Avoidant/Paranoid personality – These people are probably lurking in the background of chatrooms watching everyone else or 'flaming' (attacking) innocent email bystanders who they believe are threatening them.

Anxious/obsessional/dependent personality – They're probably meticulously organizing webpages with accurate links and multiple layers of information. These control freaks spend a lot of time communicating with all and sundry in excessive detail so that recipients come to dread receiving their messages.

Histrionic/dramatic personality – These characters have to be first in the newsgroup with the latest and greatest news. Unfortunately it's often inaccurate or exaggerated. They're constantly demanding attention from online supporters, but only contributing when they can be the focus of the group. These people aren't likely to help anyone else online unless they can tell the world about it! And if they say that they live in Hollywood, believe them!

Dissociative/multiple personality – These people are potential online disasters. If you can have multiple personalities in real life the mind boggles at what could happen online? Perhaps they could run several groups all by themselves without the need for anyone else to contribute! This would be impossibly confusing for the average online doctor.

The important point here is that the online world allows patients and therapists an extension of their normal psychological world. Whatever their normal personality or coping styles are, these are likely to be exaggerated and magnified online. This is particularly so in text only communication on the Internet where all sorts of identity fantasies can be acted out. It is common, for instance, for men to masquerade as women and to seek help for pretend disorders from online doctors; and for both sexes to act out their sexual fantasies in the "safe," but very public Internet environment. Suler provides some fascinating examples of this in his book, *The Psychology of Cyberspace*. In one example he describes how Brad met Natalie at a chatroom:

"Brad was a college senior at an eastern university, she a junior on the west coast. They got to know each other better by corresponding through email. Over time, he felt very close to her. Maybe, he thought, he was even falling in love. When he finally suggested, then insisted, that he give her a phone call, the truth came crashing down on his head. Natalie confessed to being a 50 year old man!"

Whilst this is superficially amusing, imagine how distressing it must have been for Brad. How it must have destroyed his confidence in himself.

This is an excellent example of the common social phenomenon of lying, or, as more politely defined by Jeffrey Hancock, "digital deception". There has been a lot of research into digital deception and Hancock has noted that:

"people can present in ways that they cannot in face to face encounters. Boys can be girls, the old can be young, ethnicity can be chosen, 15 year olds can be stock analysts – and on the Internet no one knows you're a dog"

Online gender deception and omitting aspects of one's identity are the most common forms of digital deception, but criminal activities are also common. The increasing number of predators on the Internet is of great concern, and is why e-practitioners should know patients names. Look at the Dateline NBC program, "To catch a predator" which focuses on online pedophiles if you don't believe this is a serious problem. Anonymity on the web in professional consultations is simply not appropriate.

THE TREATMENT PROCESS WILL CHANGE

There will be much more goal setting in eHealth which will be more goal directed than traditional treatment, and will focus more on information and education. In an ideal situation, the patient's goals will be carefully defined at the beginning of their consultation, and a treatment contract developed between the patient and the doctor to meet those goals over a defined period of time, ideally using a series of specific interventions and treatment guidelines. These will be connected to high-quality health information data bases which are easily accessible to the patient and individually tailored to their needs. The patient will be able to add to this database as they wish because increasingly our health records will be stored in such a way that they are accessible to both patients and doctors via the Internet. Many of the multinational medical records companies are already producing electronic healthcare records that can be accessed from the Internet, and the US, the UK and Australia, for example, are all introducing a national health information network which will allow all patients access to their health information. On the commercial front a number of companies, including both Microsoft and Google, have created their own personal health record platforms in partnership with academic health systems, with a view to attempting to make these more widespread across the population. This will be another major driver of a changed doctor-patient relationship - of more empowered patients. Patients are already regularly seeking other sources of help on the Internet apart from their usual face to face doctor.

Dr Andrew Lippman, the renowned futurist and viral communications expert from the Massachusetts Institute of Technology Media Lab, notes how trusting people are on the Internet, commenting that people are quite prepared to take advice from unknown Cyber-acquaintances. He uses the example of a friend of his who, needing urgent medical advice to help his child, went on the Internet, whilst his wife simultaneously phoned for the local doctor to come and see the child. On the Internet his friend discovered "Dr Flash Gordon" who said he was a doctor and emailed some simple advice to help the child. Dr Lippman said that his friend took this advice, which was accurate and helpful, and the initial crisis affecting the child was resolved even before the local doctor was able to get to his home. The back end of this story is that Dr Lippman later found out that he knew "Dr Flash Gordon"! He happened to be a colleague living in the same building! It is fascinating how his friend had been prepared to trust an unknown person with the unlikely name of "Dr Flash Gordon" on the Internet with the safety and health of his own child. There are many similar success stories of people who have used the Internet to seek help and assistance in what is essentially a global social support system. However not all health professionals welcome these situations and some doctors positively fear the changes.

A little over a hundred years ago, many doctors reacted to the advent of the telephone with hostility. They worried they'd be inundated with calls and that practicing medicine over the telephone would somehow compromise their moral integrity and promote sub-standard care. In the same way, some doctors nowadays still believe that practicing health care over the Internet is inappropriate, although almost all have their own private email addresses and use the Internet in their home lives.

In fact physicians were amongst the earliest users of the phone. The very first telephone exchange connected several Connecticut physicians to a central drug store and in the late nineteenth century telephone messages for doctors were often relayed through pharmacies. Elissa Speilberg, from Harvard Medical School, has drawn parallels between the early days of the telephone, and computer-based communications, particularly in terms of privacy and intrusiveness. She notes that "the telephone was particularly vexing to early users who complained of solicitations, eavesdroppers and even wire transmitted germs".

But by early this century doctors had learned how to screen calls and use

intermediaries to assess call priority. And, Speilberg notes, patients and doctors learned how to use the phone more effectively making patient/physician relationships "much more secure and private."

The beauty of email is that it has the potential to reach every physician, and in turn to be transmitted to all his contacts, with quite ridiculous ease. Despite this, doctors and other health care professionals have been relatively reluctant to use electronic communication in their practices, although this is changing rapidly. The reasons for this reluctance include the dread of being barraged by email and an even greater concern with privacy and confidentiality.

Interestingly doctors like me who use email regularly do not find themselves snowed under by a deluge of messages. I find it easier to respond to patients' messages at my own convenience, and often with more consideration and care, than if I was answering a telephone call on the run. I now receive far fewer phone calls because patients and clinicians I work with know that they will get a reliable reply within 24 hours by email. This is much more efficient than the past games of "telephone tag".

Reviewing the ethical considerations, Elissa Spielberg concluded *"email use suggests a profound new social dynamic within the patient/physician relationship"*. She adds that email messages: *"have the potential to be highly specific, descriptive and sometimes intimate portrayals of patient narrative and physician compassion,"* and concludes that *"email communications are not merely virtual approximations of medical practice, they are very real exchanges of information, advice and emotions"..... "The emergence of electronic communication launches a re-examination of the necessary values for good communication in the patient/physician relationship".*

If accessibility, availability and a willingness to listen are the basis of good communication between patient and physician, then email facilitates all three. Email is quick and allows patients to go into as much detail about their concerns as they wish. Those patients who are intimidated by their doctor's office or reluctant or embarrassed to detail their feelings face to face often find it much easier to be honest using the written word.

Of course in the last few years instant messaging and texting have become ubiquitous, but neither have been used to a substantial extent at the doctor-patient interface, mainly because of the likely confidentiality and privacy problems that would occur. The increased communications occurring via telephones, especially i-phones and blackberry's, make it is most likely that clinical interactions will start to occur more commonly over these modalities. Monitoring by telephone is already here, with several "health mobile phones" commercially available that will, for instance, check a blood sugar level, and automatically transmit the result to a central database.

Consumer Needs – The Era of Personalized Medicine

A number of researchers are starting to look more objectively at what are the real information needs of patients and carers, and what do they want to find when they surf the net looking for health information. And it's not what you might expect. What is valued is interactive personalized information – not necessarily the most sophisticated or most scientifically presented. People want information that relates to them, and their needs, delivered in as an immediate manner as possible, ideally through their doctor or another knowledgeable person. These needs can best be summarized as follows:

WHAT HEALTH INFORMATION DO CONSUMERS WANT FROM THE WEB?

1. Answers to my specific questions

2. Results of my searches

3. Best sites for my topic

4. Disease "guides" (see below)

5. Consumer guidelines and FAQ's (Frequently Asked Questions)

6. The ability to exchange email with my doctor, or other knowledgeable people

Equally importantly it is now understood that there are certain types of information that are generally not valued

WHAT DO CONSUMERS NOT WANT?

1. Poor quality, unreliable or biased information

2. "Shovelware"-traditional generic health information delivered pamphlet-style that is not interactive, personalized, and tends to be over-technical

3. Information that ignores the reality that most searches are performed by carers, not patients

CONSUMER GUIDES

Some good consumer-focused Websites are employing "consumer guides" or "consumer mates". One of the best known sites taking this approach is <u>www.about.com</u>. On this site, the role of a guide is described as follows:

"You're a recognized expert in your field, and you have the credentials and experience to back you up. You have professional writing experience in your area of expertise, are familiar with HTML, and love to help educate others about your topic. All guides are freelancers who work online and set their own schedules, giving them the flexibility to log on from anywhere in the world and work at a time that is best for them.

As a Guide you'll build and maintain a GuideSite, a topical section of About.com that contains:

- Original content (articles, reviews, FAQs, tutorials) written by you

- A blog featuring your unique voice and personality

- A directory of the best content on your topic, whether it is work created by you or links to other sites

- A discussion forum where you serve as community leader "

Consumer guides in the health field are frequently patients who have had an illness that is a focus of the Website and who work in partnership with the website itself, using their personal knowledge of the illness, and their extensive knowledge of the Website, to literally guide other patients to information that is appropriate for them, as well as to conduct forums, and write blogs. Such guides may provide biographies of themselves, allowing you email to them direct, tell them a bit about yourself and your health problem, and they then email back and forth with you, suggesting information on the site, and possibly on other sites, that is appropriate for you. Guides on many sites are accredited by the site and generally appear to be motivated by their wish to help others survive the illness that they themselves have had. Consumers can get the best of both worlds in this situation. They are able to link directly with another consumer who is an information expert, whilst at the same time, being literally guided round the site. This combination of consumer guides taking people around high quality reliable websites appears to me to be unbeatable. Let's hope we see much more of it in the future.

DIGGING UP INFORMATION FOR YOUR DOCTOR

Some doctors can be quite threatened by patients who have discovered a large amount of information about their health, particularly from Internet sources. While many doctors are interested in what you have found, acknowledging that you may have more time to chase up unusual sources of information than they have, others respond with confusion or bluster or in a dismissive or paternalistic manner - particularly doctors who are either ignorant of Internet health resources or who assume that such sources are inaccurate.

Others respond competitively. They take your information and rush off to the Internet themselves to prove they can find more sources than you can. Or they simply refuse to acknowledge that Internet material is valid. Fortunately these last reactions are becoming less common.

So how do you approach your doctor if you have found what looks like useful information on the Internet?

First, tell your doctor that you are Internet literate and that you intend to search for information about your problem, or that you have already made such searches. Acknowledge that there is both good and bad information on the Internet and ask your doctor to help you judge the quality and reliability of the information that you have found. Explain the search strategy you intend to use. You may find that your doctor is willing to learn that from you, as few doctors in the past were trained to search systematically, although this has now generally become a routine part of medical student education in recent years. They may well wish to follow your advice for their own purposes! Suggest you write a summary of the information that you have obtained and email this to your doctor before your visit. This is much better than presenting the poor person with hundreds of pages of downloaded information which they are highly unlikely to find time to read. Also ask your doctor for particularly good websites or other sources for your searches that they may recommend. They will frequently have a list of sites that they have looked at themselves, or that other patients have discussed with them.

Searching the Internet and other on-line resources for valuable health information can be very time consuming, and a collaborative effort with your doctor is the best way to go. Neither you, nor your doctor, can possibly know everything that is going on of relevance to your situation but there is no reason why you and your family should not be capable of becoming research assistants and librarians to help your cause. Your research can then be used by you and your doctor to develop a joint management plan to assist you.

The following is an example of an email interaction between me and the parent of one of my patients.

Dear Dr Y – I found out about the possible use of fish oil for Miranda from <u>www.schizophrenia.com</u>. There is another interesting site discussing Omega-3 fatty acids which seem to be the helpful element in the oil at <u>www.nimh.gov</u> . Can you follow up and see what you think so that we can discuss it when you next see Miranda? Thanks, John.

My reply.

Thanks John – I have emailed the psychiatrist who is doing most of the research on fish oil and described Miranda's situation to him. Attached is a copy of our correspondence. He felt it would be worth giving Miranda a go on fish oil, given her continuing symptoms and only partial response to other medications. As you know there are no guarantees, but it seems worth trying. You can buy it at most chemists as long as you tell them the seemingly active ingredient. I will find out something about dosing. Best wishes Dr Y..

Dr Y – Thanks for your answer. I have discussed this with Miranda. You will need to ask her to take the fish oil as well – you know how much a typical teenager trusts her parents on things like medication!!! Will see you next week. Regards John

Incidentally, www.schizophrenia.com, founded and run by Brian Chiko in California in memory of his brother John, who had schizophrenia, is a great example of a very well managed and successful consumer focused website. If you, or a member of your family has schizophrenia, I would certainly suggest bookmarking this in your favorites.

BLOWING THE COVER ON TECHNO-SPEAK

Doctors are famous for their technical jargon (and indecipherable writing, which online technology may now finally make comprehensible to patients!). Two good examples of medical techno-speak are dysdiadochokinesis - to flip the hand backwards and forwards quickly; and iatrogenesis - the artificial causation of a disorder by health intervention!

Acronyms make the situation worse. Did you know that in a medical record the notation "NBI" can mean either "No Bone Injury" or "No Bloody Idea", while NAD can be "No Abnormality Detected" or "Not Actually Done"!

Now add the dreadful jargon of the information and computing environment. Terms like "RAM (random access memory)" "legacy systems" (out of date systems that we can't afford to replace), "interconnectivity"(we'd love them to link, they should, but not always unfortunately), "closed systems"(can only be accessed by skilled hackers) and "best of breed" (the latest, greatest, and probably most expensive)! And this is just a sample. Actually, a lot people who use these terms don't understand them themselves but fear they will appear stupid if they ask their meanings! I have to admit I felt that way when I first got involved in information technology some years ago. Today, though, if there's a term I don't understand, I ask. This way if the person using the term knows what it means I get an explanation (and several thankful nods from people around me!) and if they don't, then I treat everything else they say with some caution.

You should always be able to understand what your online doctor is talking about. If you don't, ask!

A Note on "Netiquette"

It is crucial to communicate respectfully and professionally on the Internet, just as in life, particularly if you are emailing your doctor who is likely to be busy, and may not be forgiving if receiving inappropriate or over-casual communications. Network netiquette, or Netiquette, is simply the customs and practices which guide the behavior of Internet users. It is the online equivalent of good social behavior, the ability to smile at people, shake their hand and look them in the eye when you talk to them. Unfortunately, many people do not practice good netiquette, perhaps because of the anonymity, yet immediacy, of the Web, but also through thoughtlessness. So what are the basic rules of Netiquette?

1. Firstly, apply the same standards you follow in real life to your behavior online. My standard is to treat other people in the same way I would expect to be treated.

2. Familiarize yourself with any particular policies or procedures that might be defined by websites you are searching, or individuals you are emailing. Some sites, for instance, specifically ask you to register, and to work through a series of processes, to obtain what you wish. What's wrong with going along with their request? This is particularly important when it comes to contacting individuals by email. As an example of this, I regularly get asked to review academic papers, or be interviewed by students or journalists on email. I much prefer a polite note initially asking me if this is possible, and laying out broadly what will be expected of me, and I am generally quite positive and receptive about such requests. A significant group of individuals, however, simply send me either huge attachments to read and comment on, or even worse, multiple questions that they want me to answer, without every asking if this might be convenient or possible. When they follow up each week for

several weeks afterwards demanding to know why I haven't done it, if I haven't, my blood pressure rises rapidly.

3. Think of other people's time, of the bandwidth you are using, and the storage space you may be taking up. We simply cannot continue to use email in an exponential manner and there is a tendency for people to send large attachments around to many folk just because it's easy. Especially in this day where video clips are so easily available. So send the link to the video file instead of the whole file, or put the file you want to share on a website, and then send the link. I have done quite a lot of work on virtual reality, for instance, and often want to show people video examples, so I have uploaded some video clips to my professional site at the Department of Psychiatry at UC Davis, (www.ucdmc.ucdavis.edu/psychiatry) but have also put some clips on youtube.comIf you search with my name you will find them easily. Equally, emails with fancy multimedia logos or signatures take up large amounts of room on computers. I already very regularly have to clean up the memory on my computer, and much of it is taken up by irrelevant files that have been received on email.

4. Be polite. If you get flamed, the chances are you have broken the rules of netiquette. Unfortunately, "flamewars" easily break out when many people start sending flames to each other. These are not only very upsetting for the individuals involved, and for observers, but clearly also congest the network.

5. Try to avoid "SHOUTING". The convention of the Internet is that capital letters are used expressively to show angry feelings. Apart from the fact that letters in upper case are often more difficult to read, you need to be aware of this convention.

6. If you are writing to somebody, then do them the courtesy of including a descriptive header in your message. I can assure you that, once you start getting 100-200 emails a day, as happens to me, you become very intolerant of people who don't tell you why they are contacting you! Even though my university runs great spam filters, and does its best to prevent intrusion by viruses, unless I know who has emailed me, I routinely delete all email without clear understandable headers.

7. Respect other people's privacy. Privacy is as important on the online world, as it is in the real world. So only contact people if you really think it is necessary. Generally contact which includes abuse in any form, particularly poor language, or racist and sexist remarks, the sending

of chain letters, broadcasting messages to massive lists, or actions which interfere with the work of other people are seen as breaches of netiquette.

EMOTICONS

It is still difficult to fully show one's emotions when using email to interact. It is, however, possible to use a series of what are called "emoticons" that have evolved over the last few years by convention, on the web, to identify your emotional state to your receiver. Equally, as instant messaging has evolved the whole language and spelling of regular messaging users has changed - ask anybody under 25 years old to explain the shortcuts! The following list of emoticons are examples –

: -)	User is happy	: - x	User's lips are sealed
: - (	User is sad	# -)	User partied all night
: - t	User is cross	: - 0	User is shocked

THE EMAIL RELATIONSHIP.

Deciding whether to have long term or ongoing consultations by email is a major decision. Often you will write in great depth and length, with passion, confusion, anger or joy. It is somewhat like writing a diary except that the diary can write back! And of course, the diary that does write back is a blog (derived from web-log). Most problems are quite complex and are not likely to be resolved overnight. It will take some time for you and your doctor or therapist to trust each other and to develop a therapeutic alliance or relationship. You need to be prepared to enter into a process of change and be honest with yourself and your doctor. All of this is much easier if your online doctor is also your face to face doctor, and your email consultations are of the type 2 variety. Way back in 1998 Dr Tom Ferguson MD correctly predicted what would happen in terms of the email and broader online relationship between patients and their doctor:

"Physicians may find it far easier than they think to offer their patients their own personalized blend of highly accessible, high quality, online health resources. In addition to welcoming patient email under appropriate circumstances, physicians might establish their own Web pages with lists of frequently asked patient questions and answers and annotated links to useful and authoritative medical Websites. Physicians could also provide biographical information, explain their practice philosophy, offer online appointment scheduling, and point to high quality health data bases and directories of online support groups. Such resources could serve

current patients, help attract new ones, and might even allow physicians to budget their own time more effectively. Clinicians who invite their patients to join them in electronic conversation may reap another benefit as well – a better appreciation for the "other" side of their patient/physician relationship, which has commanded increased attention and has come under increased pressure under recent years."

There are three criteria for a successful email relationship - you feel comfortable using email and the Internet, you have the time for, and enjoy, writing and you can write honestly and expressively about your feelings and reactions.

Dr Ellen Rothchild MD, a past Chairperson of the American Psychiatric Association Telemedical Committee, comments on patient-doctor communication by email.

It *"holds promises and pitfalls. Email can be edited, printed and filed. Time zones and hearing and speech impediments become irrelevant. One message can go to many recipients. An emotionally needy patient with low tolerance for frustration in between appointments may be encouraged to email thoughts between visits as an alternative to frequent phoning. Email, like web-surfing, can be exciting in its novelty and potential."*

John Suler, in his online book "Psychology of Cyberspace" looks at several other important issues relating to the way we communicate online: *"When we are on the Internet we all tend to regress and act in a more child like manner. We tend to be less inhibited and more likely to act in primitive ways, in particular by "flaming" - attacking others who are online".*

The first online list I ever joined, for instance, which had been set up for health professionals only, demonstrated this perfectly. A person with differing political views from others on the list was flamed unmercifully and cruelly. By the time the list moderator tried to intervene, it was too late. Some very hurtful things had been said which would certainly not have been said face to face. The result was that many people, including myself, resigned from the list.

Sexual harassment is also unfortunately very common on the net. This is why you should be quite sure your online friends are who they say they are before you reveal any personal details. Despite all this I am continually amazed at the lengths people go to help each other and by the remarkable generosity and warmth shown by so many to complete strangers, especially in chat rooms and on discussion lists. The anonymity and asynchronous interaction of the net may cause further problems. Because we can't see the person sending the message, and because they can use pseudonyms and addresses at Internet Service Providers, it is very difficult to identify individuals who want to remain anonymous. This anonymity amplifies the disinhibiting effect of email and can be good or bad depending on whether people are excessively rude or warm.

Email conversations don't usually occur in real time. They can take place over hours, weeks or even months. The advantage of this is that doctors and patients have more time to consider and evaluate their responses than in other therapeutic situations. When I receive emails that annoy me, unless they are very urgent, I deliberately wait a day or so before answering. A considered reply is generally more valuable than an immediate one. Email communication means plans and goals can be carefully designed, considered and reconsidered to achieve the best therapeutic outcome instead of everything being squeezed into a single, often rushed, consultation.

Using email, people can receive health education individually or in any size of groups through open or closed chatrooms, secure or public spaces or lists, bulletin boards or support groups. One clinical educator can interact with many patient "students." Group work and information dissemination has been greatly enhanced through easily downloadable videos using "video streaming" techniques, such as from www.youtube.com, and numerous other video sites. A number of sites now offer Video mail – video letters, while others encourage users to send in still or video files. The best general example of this is the I-reports at cnn.com. Similarly online medical journals are changing substantially led by the Medscape Journal of Medicine (www.medscape.com) which now routinely presents Web Video Editorials. These are peer-reviewed high quality short editorials written by guest editors of the Journal, which are presented in full video format, with the writers presenting their papers in video clips that typically last about 3 minutes. It is so much easier to "watch" an editorial, than to have to read it all, and very helpful to "see" the presenter, rather than just read their words. The Medscape video clips are also made available to the general public on youtube.com and Google video. I have done several of these if you want to look. Major health corporations have long worked out the potential cost savings of providing online multi-party health education - estimated to take as much as 20% of typical expensive medical outpatient time – and almost all health institutions now offer substantial educational material for patients via their websites.

PATIENTS EMBRACING CHANGE

There is no doubt that online technology will mean radical changes for both doctors and patients. But what do patients think about this? I've found patients are not concerned about being interviewed or treated online. Let's face it, people who are used to watching shows by Jerry Springer or Oprah Winfrey are hardly going to be upset by the prospect of "seeing" their doctor on a computer.

My experience is that patients often feel that eHealth is more private than, say, a hospital ward where they may be asked intimate details of their personal and sexual life with only a curtain between them and several other patients!

In further evidence of patient acceptance Dr Warner Slack has described how over a five and a half year period 2,500 employees took part in computer interviews on their lifestyles at the Beth Israel hospital in Boston. And the survey results - 57% of the employees reported high levels of stress, 43% reported feeling "sad, discouraged or hopeless" in the previous month, while 6% indicated that "life sometimes did not feel worth living". 85% of the participants responded positively to the computer interview and when asked to compare the computer-based interview with an interview with a doctor or nurse, most participants preferred the computer.

In further studies Dr Slack discovered that patients being treated for alcoholism also found it easier to report high levels of alcohol consumption to a computer than to a psychiatrist while others were more likely to reveal sexual problems, a criminal record, impotence, being fired from a job or even suicide attempts to a computer rather than a person.

The final word on email relationships should go to Gary Stofle (www. stofle.com) a social worker who started providing email psychotherapy in 1996, and who retired from this component of his practice in 2008, but who has reflected on his learnings:

"We can provide psychotherapy online. Human beings are wonderfully adaptable. We have found many wonderful and unusual ways of communicating with one another. For centuries we have used the written word to express thoughts, feelings and opinions with one another. We have used the written word to titillate, to persuade, to con, manipulate and harm others. And we have also used the written word to heal. Online psychotherapy is a way ethical therapists can use the written word to heal through establishing a therapeutic relationship."

To summarize:

- The doctor-patient relationship has two main components – empathy and expertise

- Information rich patients will increasingly drive the doctor-patient relationship

- Transference, counter transference, and our personality characteristics are all important online, where good "netiquette" is crucial

- The era of personalized medicine will include an increased focus on good online communication between patients and doctors – good online netiquette is of great importance.

8

Telephobia, Tele-Addiction And Cyberchondria

Nothing in life is free of risks and the Internet is no exception. Especially where health is concerned. Most of the time the risks are really just to do with poor information or advice, and the tips in this book will help with them. Even dishonest relationships can usually be identified, although sometimes too late to prevent damage.

POTENTIAL RISKS FOR PATIENTS ON THE WEB

- Internet addiction – excess dependence on the virtual world

- Poor advice, especially from anonymous chat rooms

- Poor quality information

- Financial loss – through payment to poorly trained therapists, or for unproven therapies or health products

- Dishonest relationships where one or other partner in a relationship is deceitful about who they are, what they do, or what they wish

However there are some specific syndromes that are increasingly being recognized by doctors and Internet researchers which merit special attention. Despite our move to cyberspace, many people are still scared of technology.

That's telephobia. On the other hand, some people can't get enough of it …… that's tele-addiction! And some people just go overboard in their worry about symptoms they have read about on the net – that's cyberchondria!

TELEPHOBIA

Despite living in the "information age" it is a recognized fact that more than half of us are frightened by technology! Ask yourself… can you program your video? Sure, we can all turn them on and off and do simple recordings but anything more demanding, well! And mobile phones…even the touch phones at home! There dozens of different varieties that can be bought, from the iPhone and Blackberry to phones of almost every color, size and complexity. How many people do you know who use all, or even most of the options? Is it that we are too lazy, disinterested, too busy …. or too afraid to work them out? And if we're baffled by mobile phones and video recorders, how much more disconcerting are computers and other hi-tech equipment for some people.

Really, we only need to know as much about the technology as is required to accomplish our tasks. Of course, if we suddenly decide it's much more interesting than we thought, we can always go further…. learn more tricks and techniques, use more software. But for most of us, it's just a matter of learning the basics of what we need. Forget about trying to work out what makes them tick. After all when we buy cars and lawnmowers we don't make their service manuals bedside reading. For some reason, most people think computers are different.

We all respond differently to new technologies but for many of us they bring on a feeling of "technostress". According to Californian psychologists, Dr Michelle Weil PhD and Dr Larry Rosen PhD technostress is:

> *"the irritation we feel as our boundaries are constantly invaded by beeps, pagers and cell phone conversations……..It is our feeling that we should be able to work as fast as our computers. It is our bewilderment that with so many time-saving devices, we never have enough time. Technostress is our feeling of helplessness when our children or neighbors can 'surf the web' and we still do not know what that means!"*

These sorts of stresses can lead to technophobias and telephobias. In his book, "Technophobia" Mark Brosnan describes Technophobia as:

> *"a resistance to talking about computers or even thinking about computers, fear or anxiety towards computers, hostile or aggressive thoughts about computers"*

Many people still don't like the idea that computers are now part and parcel of our lives…. like it or not, online technology is all around us….. we will all have to become involved and have some understanding of it. People with telephobia react to their often unconscious fear of the technology often turn round and shoot the messenger. They complain that it won't do what it's supposed to do, that the equipment isn't good enough and, in the case of many clinicians, that the patients won't like it. Many doctors also fear the changes to their practices that online technology will bring.

Fear of being online is usually associated with computers…but not exclusively. If you are the victim of a stalker, are receiving crank phone calls or expecting bad news you may dread the telephone ringing. You may even refuse to answer it. I have seen patients in these situations who have become completely phobic about phones. One woman I knew eventually decided to do away with her telephone altogether. She associated phones with such dreadful news and distress that even having one in her home and office made her anxious. It certainly made her job as an architect more difficult but she solved the problem by using a messenger service to deliver handwritten letters between her clients and friends and herself. Luckily, her friends were very understanding. Sadly there have been many cases of "stalking," or harassment, on the Internet. The stalkers posted personal details and addresses of their victims on the net, usually suggesting the person was available for sexual favors. This is a particular risk on social networking sites where your new "friend" may not be so friendly. Fortunately some of these criminals have now been jailed, but it would hardly be surprising if their victims became afraid of computers after such a frightening experience.

In "Technophobia" Mark Brosnan suggests technophobia is a legitimate response to technology and that this fear of technology is caused by social and cultural factors inherent in our society. Maybe it is a sense of social shame at their computer illiteracy that has led to thousands of American senior managers attending very expensive short courses in basic computing often at secret exotic locations. Even now, in 2008, I know of some senior executives who literally cannot log on, although they are becoming few and far between.

It has also been suggested that telephobia is related to old age, and to a degree that is true. However as over 35% of people over 65 now use the Internet or email regularly and over 70% of those in the 50-65 year old age group are actively online, this is more likely to be a generational issue. This is particularly important as elderly people will benefit enormously from online homecare.

WE EITHER LOVE IT OR HATE IT!

We all tend to fall into three distinct groups in our reaction to technology…... Rosen and Weil describe us as "eager adopters", "hesitant 'prove its'" and "resisters". Which are you?

"Eager adopters"

They love the technology. They view online activities as challenging and fun. They are always the first people to buy the latest technologies, and they love experimenting and treat new technologies like new toys. I am one of these! Typically, I don't expect the technology to always be perfect, or even work and I don't blame myself when it doesn't! The "eager adopters" include "nerds", computer salesmen and technology enthusiasts. A lot of doctors are among this group. They tend to get heavily involved in the relatively new disciplines of health informatics and telemedicine. If you are interested in these areas look at the websites from the American Medical Informatics Association (www. amia.org) and the American Telemedicine Association (www.atmeda.org) . Although this group of early adopters only makes up 10% of the population, most marketing is directed at it, as this is the group that will kick start sales of any interesting novel technology. Not surprisingly, in the technology field, this group is dominated by young men, as you will find if you go to any technology innovation conference.

"Hesitant 'prove its'"

Most people fall into this group…. about 60-80% of the population. They don't see online activities as much fun and only get involved when it can be clearly demonstrated that the activities are worthwhile. They're not into experimenting or sorting out their own online difficulties… preferring to call in help! Once convinced, however, this group rapidly become heavy users of new technologies – just look at how ubiquitously email has been adopted at home and in the workforce over the past 15 years. What would we do without it? Very few people, once they start using email or the Internet, give up and go back to letter writing. This is the group which will get a lot of use out of eHealth as long they concentrate on what they need and don't get bogged down with the technical side. People in this group are potential telephobics if they have bad experiences or don't receive the training they need. But their telephobias are eminently treatable. Most women fall into this category.

The "Resisters"

Comprising about 10% of the population, this group avoids technology as much as possible! Technology intimidates them. They tend to blame themselves when problems arise and this increases their feelings of inadequacy and fuels their determination to avoid online technology in the future. To cover their underlying anxiety they tend to attack the technology. Some even proudly call themselves "computer luddites" or "techno-luddites."

How many of the following statements apply to you?

• I do not feel confident about operating a computer at a basic level.

• I am not interested in computer shops or product displays.

• I would not post an anonymous personal comment on an Internet bulletin board.

• I would not be prepared to email my usual doctor.

• I use the phone for necessary conversations only and do not like spending much time on it.

• I believe that information technology is greatly overrated in our society.

• Given the choice of a session on the Internet or a cold shower, I would choose the shower.

• I believe that the spread of information technology is a global attempt by big business to take over the world to satisfy their need to be in control.

• I do not like the idea of having a computer in my home.

• I will not enter a credit card number onto the Internet even if the site is meant to be secure.

If you agreed with four or more of the above, you may well be telephobic.

OK, I AM TELEPHOBIC...WHAT CAN I DO ABOUT IT?

The best way to conquer a fear is to acknowledge that it exists, learn about it and then confront it. Some years ago I spoke to a shark hunter. I asked him how he'd become involved in such an unusual occupation. His reply was that for years he'd been terrified of sharks and this was the only way to overcome this fear. Admittedly, his story is somewhat extreme!

There are two ways of overcoming telephobia…. As a community, we need to change the way the technologies are presented so that they are more user-friendly and relevant. On a personal level people may need to seek individualized help for specific problems. But first let's look at the causes of telephobia.

MALE BIASES

Many more females than males are telephobic and it only takes a glance at the whole computer culture to see why. From an early age boys show more interest in computers – perhaps because computer store shelves are stacked with shooting, killing games which target males. In contrast there are less games that appeal to girls.

Technology advertising targets men. Do a Google search for "social marketing" or "social media solutions" and see what comes up. An astonishing industry focused on social and gender manipulation. Look at this annonymized description of what is often called "behavioral targeting":

"Behavioral targeting offers advertisers the opportunity to expand the reach and frequency of their online campaigns and engage their target audience. Our advanced behavioral targeting gives advertisers the ability to find users who are actively seeking information about their products or services throughout the purchase cycle: awareness, information search, alternative evaluation, purchase decision and post-purchase behavior. Advertisers can target these audience segments with specific messaging tailored for each stage in order to maximize relevance and strengthen brand awareness."

Most technology marketing is based on the computer's power or its social trendiness. Macintosh argues that it is a younger more hip brand than PC's. And computers are sold on the basis of the size of their RAM - Random Access Memory – the bigger and more powerful the better …. the parallel with the penis is exquisitely overt! What about the size of your 'hard drive'? - no comment! Is your broadband connection fast enough to crash through the superhighway? Maybe the advertising gurus who dream up these slogans and macho advertising techniques don't realize that women may receive, often unconsciously, the reverse messages of rape and disempowerment. It is not surprising so many women distrust technology.

Paradoxically, women actually use computers more than men because of the predominance of women in secretarial roles. And they have been the leaders in the social networking phenomenon of the past few years. The last statistics I could find on facebook usage showed that there were 42 million users around the world in November 2007, and 27 million of these were females.

Brosnan is in no doubt that the information industry's masculine bias is socially, not biologically, determined which he says, *"can make computing motivationally problematic for feminine individuals (whether male or female)".*

Women are not the only group in society under-represented in the computer industry – on a population basis African-Americans and Latinos are also under-represented, while Asians are significantly over-represented. And in terms of users, we know that the most important single social issue that leads to underuse of computer technology is poverty. So whenever you find poverty, such as in rural Tulare County in California, the poorest county in the whole of the US, you will find relatively low levels of computer literacy, whether the population is Caucasian, Latino, African-American or Asian. And as you move outside the US, the digital divide, driven by poverty and geography, is of course more severe in underdeveloped countries, especially in Africa.

HOW CHANGING THE COMPUTER INDUSTRY WOULD HELP PREVENT TELEPHOBIA

Feminizing The Industry and Changing The Culture: This is important and is beginning to happen. Until the masculine bias in the computer industry changes it will be hard to prevent many of the telephobic symptoms experienced by females. Girls as well as boys need to feel comfortable with computers from an early age. We need more computer software that interests girls. There needs to be a change in the attitude of teachers and in the content of courses in computing and information technology to make the subjects more appealing to females. There needs to be more females in senior positions in the IT industry. Carly Fiorini, the ex-CEO of Hewlett-Packard, is one of very few females who have broken the glass ceiling in this industry.

Changing the product and the marketing: The industry needs to identify a need and then design the product to fill it. At present the industry is infamous for its tendency to develop a new "toy" and then search out a market or a use for it - putting the cart before the horse. This is commonly associated with the approach of "build it and they will come". More market research needs to be carried out on how our lifestyles could be enhanced by the technology. Our needs should determine what products are created. The 90% percent of us who are not "eager adopters" simply need computers which fulfill our basic requirements. Warner Slack MD sums up the situation perfectly...."*When* *computer manufacturers ask 'How can we get physicians to use computers' they are more likely to mean 'How can we get physicians to buy computers?' A better question would be 'How can we make our computers more helpful"*

More collaboration and social conscience: The big players, such as Microsoft, Google Intel, Cisco, Macintosh and the like, need to develop a stronger social conscience, working together to use technological advances for social gain. (Less importance could be attached to market domination and obscene executive salaries). When did you last see a multinational information technology company promoting social advantage as being as important as profits? While they all have foundations, ultimately companies are responsible to shareholders, and these are the people who can make them change. This is starting to happen as major investors, such as retirement funds, increasingly challenge companies to have strong social consciences. Jack Ehnes, CEO of the California State Teachers Retirement System, with billions of dollars invested in major companies has been particularly strong on insisting that companies are environmentally careful. In 2004 he was quoted describing the performance of an oil pipeline company as saying " reporting on greenhouse gas emissions is good for business and good for the planet."

Socially responsible computer education programs: Currently computer education programs seem designed to produce propeller heads whose only desire is to write new programs or invent bizarre incomprehensible acronyms. Of course this computer jargon is a great way of excluding non-members. We still know very little about the effects of computers and particularly the Internet, on society although there is a massive amount of research in the early stages. What we need are education programs which concentrate on what the market needs and how the products affect society. Such programs are as important as the technological advances themselves.

ANOTHER CHANGE. THE HEALTH INDUSTRY SHOULD BE GREENER

Healthcare is the second largest energy consumer of all industrial sectors, but has a poor environmental record with only about 2% of US healthcare construction judged as green. A story in Newsweek in 2008 summarized the Presidential candidates' policies on the environment and concluded that, whoever is elected leader later in the year, it is likely that they will develop a comprehensive energy plan with conservation as an essential component. A recent medical review by Paul Auerbach MD described the environment as "today's most pressing global issue". Isn't it ironic that the health industry, comprising thousands of people dedicated to improving health, is at the bottom rank of industries in terms of its environmental policies. As health professionals, in this area, we literally do make our patients, and ourselves, sick.

More than 50% of the total energy consumption in healthcare is used for heating and cooling, with annual costs averaging $3.71 per square foot. The US Environmental Protection Agency (www.epa.gov) estimates that 3.4 billion pounds of solid waste is produced each year by US hospitals with more than 50% in the form of paper and cardboard. At UC Davis, which is an energy conscious hospital with active recycling and energy conservation programs, we have calculated that for each patient admitted as an inpatient we use the equivalent energy of 240 gallons of gas – enough to drive across the USA and back again. This is an extraordinary amount of energy per admission, but is probably much less than many hospitals. Healthcare is a mobile industry, as well as one that maintains large numbers of buildings. Each gallon of fuel consumed while driving results in about 20 pounds of carbon dioxide pollution in the atmosphere. This is approximately 1.7 billion tons each year in the US. Clinicians and patients are responsible for much of this as they drive long distances to meet, have tests, and undertake interventions.

As healthcare professionals it is evident that we are contributing in our daily work to an unhealthy planet, and creating a worse environment for ourselves, our patients, and future generations. We need to change the way we practice medicine and substantially reduce the amount of travel and paper associated with our work in order to protect our environment. We can do this through increasing the use of telemedicine and electronic communications technologies like email.

We know that telemedicine saves large amounts of travel for patients and clinicians. In the past this has been seen primarily as a positive cost and time benefit. In future it will be seen as an essential conservation practice as we move to a time where we may receive "carbon credits" for increased electronic health activity.

This is a strong argument to increase the use of telemedicine, email, and telephony to communicate with our patients, and to further implement electronic medical records and electronic prescribing. From a conservation perspective we should treat more people in their homes or work sites using Internet based chronic disease management programs, self-care approaches and patient owned or accessed personal health records. We also need to increase the use of electronic systems for education and research, and take a digitally driven preventative and public health approach to delivering population based care and biosurveillance. A well planned digital world will be better for our environment, our patients and our families, and will encourage more people to use technology appropriately.

HELPING OURSELVES

Sadly it's unrealistic to believe that the computer culture, never mind the health culture, will change overnight. We still have to cope with our own fears and problems, and the following three broad approaches, used either individually, or together, generally work.

1. Give yourself time.

You can't become comfortable with online technology overnight. As in any new situation it takes time to adapt and feel at ease. When we don't give ourselves enough time our natural defense is to either fight or flee. We end up either getting angry with the technology, calling it "useless" or something much stronger, or running away! Either is an effective short-term response to our anxiety but doesn't do much for our long-term goal of learning to go online.

2. Obtain tuition using adult learning principles

We all learn best when given specific problems to solve in a supportive environment where non-judgmental help is readily available. For example if you want to learn how to send email, the aim of the first teaching session should be to successfully send a simple email. Don't waste your time trying to understand what makes the computer work or the theory behind sending emails! Simply focus on how to accomplish the task. The extra "bells and whistles' can be covered in follow up sessions. Countless people have been turned off using these technologies by being told to "sit down and get on with it… anyone can do it". This approach is a recipe for disaster. Thankfully the boring software manuals of the past have been replaced with far more user-friendly onscreen "help" icons and multimedia video presentations. And more education programs are online, either free or available on a commercial basis, so it is always worthwhile looking for multimedia presentations if you want to pick up new skills quickly and easily.

3. Anxiety reduction programs can help.

These programs use desensitization techniques to help phobic users relax when using a computer, or other technology, while at the same time allowing the individuals' time to experiment safely online in a supportive situation. A fear response is replaced by a relaxation response. If you think an anxiety reduction program could help you, then Brosnan's book "Technophobia" contains some sensible advice. Alternatively consult a therapist for a straightforward treatment program.

TELE-ADDICTION

At the opposite end of the spectrum from the telephobics are the Tele- addicts! They are the stuff of computer salesmen's dreams! While "Tele-Addiction" doesn't yet appear in the American Psychiatric Association's Diagnostic and Statistical Manual of Psychiatric Disorders, there is a move to have it included. It is also referred to as Problematic Internet Use, Computer Addiction, Internet Addiction Disorder, Pathological Computer Use, Technosis and Cyberspace Addiction. Rather paradoxically there are a number of Internet support groups for "addicts".

Most people in western societies will have read of cases of Internet addiction or know of people afflicted symptoms. There are always some people who will go overboard with any new experience. While the online world provides a welcome escape for many people, taken to the extreme it can affect normal social activity, family relationships and psychological development. While most people believe that being online relieves loneliness, this may not be the case for everyone. A study from Carnegie Mellon University found that individuals who spent even a few hours each week online experienced greater levels of depression and loneliness than if they had spent less time on the computer! The researchers hypothesized that relationships maintained over long distances without face to face contact ultimately do not provide the kind of support that makes us feel secure and happy. Friends on the Internet aren't available to baby-sit at short notice, or have a cup of coffee. However they felt the Internet could be very successful in maintaining ties with friends who lived close by. Maybe it's just when we spend a lot of time keeping up relationships with people who live too far away for us to see much that we run into problems. The evidence isn't in on this issue yet and more research programs are being undertaken, but do take care and don't assume that the Internet is all good.

There is substantial evidence that most computer addicts are males. Some researchers have gone so far as to suggest that it is only males who identify intimately with computers! This may seem far-fetched but, if true, the implications are mind boggling. Does this mean that males attach female characteristics to their computers and that the huge number of pornographic sites on the web is proof of the computers sexuality?! Or are socially avoidant males having relationships with asexual computer "mates" who have identical interests! It's probably safe to assume if you have assigned your computer a name and personality you are showing signs of tele-addiction.

Advice columnists and other "agony aunts" receive many letters a week from women and men who seek wondering whether to leave their spouse for someone they have met on the net. It is no longer uncommon for people to meet their spouses online. Many of these people will have isolated themselves in what Michelle Weil and Larry Rosen call their own "techno-cocoon", distancing themselves from the family unit. Of course, technology is not always the cause of the problem. The problem may be already there, and the net relationship just a symptom. Someone who feels isolated in the family unit may be drawn to the comfort of the Internet, further alienating themselves from their family and social system.

Internet activities are especially addictive. Surfing the net is rather like going fishing – one always expects to find the ultimate webpage in the next few minutes, just like one hopes to catch the largest fish in the river. When we do find a great website, possibly after hours of surfing frustration, our gambling instincts are reinforced and we carry on looking for the next "big win". Email users often have a tendency to check their mail several times a day - "just in case". Evidence is now emerging that email may interfere with work and home efficiency, and enjoyment of life, if it is not carefully managed. I am a good example of someone who receives a lot of email; from patients, colleagues and researchers, and friends from all over the world. Whilst it is great to stay in touch it can take up a lot of my day and I've had to rearrange my work so that I don't spend all my evenings on the computer and never see my family. And unfortunately I'm not always successful!

Virtual reality games, particularly those seen in arcades, are also addictive. They are carefully designed to appeal to the competitive element in us all. We have to continuously aim for higher levels of play, perform harder tricks, shoot more people or score more points. And while the games constantly reward success, very few people actually reach the highest levels.

On top of addictions some of these games cause symptoms of the "post simulator syndrome." For instance, users of flight simulators sometimes experience illusions of turning or difficulty walking after a prolonged "ride" on the simulator. These symptoms can be so common that armed forces pilots are often actually restricted from flying real airplanes for between 12 and 24 hours after "flying" a simulator. We know that practicing on virtual reality three dimensional games before a session of robotic minimally invasive surgery can improve surgeon's manual dexterity and literally "warm them up" so that they operate more accurately, and that the best surgeons in this field tend to also be very good at computer games! As long as they don't go overboard, computer games in the operating room make sense, but there will likely be a requirement to restrict driving or operating heavy machinery for a few hours after being in a virtual environment in future.

How Do You Recognize a Tele-Addict?

Addictions are simply behaviors over which we have little control. They can cause us distress or disrupt our lives personally or socially. It is easy to see how this can happen in cyberspace. Many of us will know people who have become tele-addicted. You may even be a tele-addict yourself. The desperate wife of an addict recently posted this note on the Internet:

"I'm so angry with all of you out there. You've taken my husband from me. He won't talk to us anymore because he lives in a fantasy land – the same fantasy land that you're all in!!!! Snap out of it! Live your lives and speak to people face to face. He doesn't think there's a problem. He's on all night – he doesn't know his family anymore. I'm so desperate I'm calling on you to reply to me so I can show him what you think and hope that he wakes up to himself. He might believe something you say cos he won't believe me. I can't believe I am asking you people in cyberspace to help me get my husband back to the real world."

Dr Kimberley Young PhD published a book entitled "Caught in the Net," in which she described the following eight signs as being typical warnings of Internet addiction, and suggested that five or more positive responses may indicate addiction.

- Do you feel preoccupied with the Internet (think about previous online activity or anticipate the next online session)?

- Do you feel the need to use the Internet for increasing amounts of time in order to achieve satisfaction?

- Have you repeatedly made unsuccessful efforts to control, cut back or stop Internet use?

- Do you feel restless, moody, depressed, or irritable when attempting to cut down or stop Internet use?

- Do you stay online longer than you originally intended?

- Have you jeopardized or risked the loss of a significant relationship, job, educational or career opportunity because of the Internet?

- Have you lied to family members, therapist or others to conceal the extent of involvement with the Internet?

- Do you use the Internet as a way of escaping from problems or of relieving a dysphoric mood (feelings of helplessness, guilt, anxiety or depression)?

Young's criteria quickly took hold in the Internet research community and two camps have formed in the area of Internet research – one which feels that Internet addiction is, or should be, established as a psychiatric disorder in its own right, and one which insists that Internet addiction sufferers are actually dependent on some rewarding aspect or function of behavior associated with Internet use that could exist in the "real" world, such as dependent or addictive behavioral patterns related to money or sex. I am in the latter camp.

Those who define Internet addiction as a specific mental illness have developed most of the estimates of the prevalence of the problem, but these estimates vary greatly, from as low as 3% , to 15-25%. Researchers in the other camp have not denied the addictive features of the Internet, but generally assert that users are addicted to the material they find on the Internet, such as online gambling, shopping, or chatting, not to the medium itself. A number of differences have been found to exist between those who use the Internet in a healthy way and those who do not. Individuals found to be "Internet-dependent" have also frequently been found to be more attracted to interactive Internet applications, such as chatting, games, and shopping, whereas non-dependent individuals seem to use the Internet almost exclusively for sending email and searching for information. Young found that just over half of those labeled "Internet dependent" had been online for less than one year, indicating that new users may be more inclined to develop problematic behaviors associated with their Internet use, a finding supported by later studies.

A large proportion of individuals who overuse the Internet also have been addicted to alcohol or drugs. Perhaps most significantly, a number of researchers have identified impulse control problems in conjunction with problematic Internet use. In one study, nearly all respondents frequently felt an urge to be online, felt that a world without the Internet would be dull, and became nervous if their Internet connection was slow. Overall, it seems more likely that the content on the Internet, such as online gambling, interactive games, or chatting, is what stimulates these reward systems, rather than simply access to the Internet itself.

Whilst Young's list is serious not everyone takes Internet addictions as seriously. The following warning signs are found at Netaholics Anonymous (www.safari.net). (There **is** an element of truth in them!)

You wake at 3 a.m. to go to the bathroom and stop and check your email on the way back to bed.

You get a tattoo which reads "This body best viewed with Netscape Navigator or higher"

You name your children Eudora and Dot.com

You spend half of the plane trip with your laptop on your lap.…. .and your child in the overhead compartment.
Your hard drive crashes. You haven't logged in for two hours. You start to twitch. You pick up the phone and manually dial your Internet service providers' number. You try to hum to communicate with the modem. You succeed!!

In reality no-one knows how many people have tele-addictions or exactly who they are. Dr John Suler PhD has noted that there is a problem *"when your face to face life becomes dissociated from your cyberlife"* and notes the important corollary that *"It's healthy when your face to face life is integrated with your cyberlife."*
Posted by Newbie.
Hi, I'm new here and I have a problem. I am sixteen years old and am involved in an online relationship with a girl who lives in Michigan. Almost every day we meet in a chatroom. Then one day she didn't turn up and I got worried. She didn't respond for two weeks. I went to some of the websites she visits and posted "missing persons post" in guestbooks and message boards. I and some of my friends emailed her for two weeks but still there was no reply. Eventually she replied to say that she had gone on vacation for 2 weeks and telling me to get a life and leave her alone. She told me she had found some new friends and wasn't going to hang out on the Internet so much in future. She said she thought I should do the same. This made me think because I was so upset. I just realized that I don't have a life because I spend so much time online – like 8-12 hours per day. My family is suffering from financial and money problems and I've been turned down for jobs. My parents won't let me drive the car (insurance problems) so I basically don't go outside the house and I had nothing better to do than go online. The pain of losing her is so bad – she wants me to leave her alone and I must respect her wishes…. I feel like a tortured soul….This is tearing me up. Thanks for reading this and giving me some advice.
Reply by Anita
Hi – I can really relate to what you say. I have "dated" 4 guys off the Internet. I know it is really easy to think you have fallen in love with someone over the Internet, but trust me, it's not the same. I have even had supposed boyfriends send me pictures of them that weren't even them!! You are young. You may not like to hear this, but what she said is right. It's hard to have a normal relationship on the Internet. I am engaged to a guy I met on the net, but we agreed not to make any commitments until we met in person – that was smart and safe. And the good thing is that we both do lots of other things away from the Internet although we both still really like it. I don't think your relationship would have gone too far, and even though you've had a bad experience if you take the advice it might turn out for the best in the long run. I hope I've helped ya just a little.

Cyberchondria

This is one of the most recent words spawned by the Internet, and is a form of Internet addiction driven by anxiety. We all get somewhat hypochondriacal on occasions, and believe that we have illnesses where none exist. Patients who in the past have had "hypochondria" have tended to present to their doctors with the latest medical dictionary, or pharmaceutical book. Alternatively, they have heard tales of woe from a friend, a colleague, or the local gossip suggesting that the minor symptom that they had may be a sign of impending doom and a long and prolonged death. Medical students, for example, are well-known to worry that they have symptoms of the diseases that they study. A proportion of them regularly end up seeing dermatologists, worrying about their own spots and lesions, soon after they have studied skins, or get their eyes checked after an ophthalmology term. It's quite natural, therefore, that if we all suddenly have access to huge amounts of health information, that we might start imagining that we have dreadful illnesses. This is certainly happening. There is no doubt that some patients are presenting with symptoms of "cyberchondria". I have seen several in my own practice. "Treatment" generally consisted of providing reassuring and accurate information about their health status, and teaching them how to work together to analyze the health information that they found on the Web more critically. Having said that I have treated one young man, a very intelligent university student, who had to be literally withdrawn from the Internet because he was spending up to 18 hours per day searching for "cures" for his fantasy illnesses. Luckily he had understanding parents who did not have a computer at their home and who let him move back with them for several months so that he could be "dried out" in an Internet free environment!

Preventing or Treating the Addiction

Information about the treatment and prevention of tele-addictions is thin on the ground, presumably because they have only recently been recognized. If you search on Google you will immediately find a number of counseling sites that offer treatment – both online and potentially on an inpatient basis. I am deliberately not identifying any particular programs in this book, because this is such a controversial area. Other countries are taking a more aggressive approach, particularly in the Asian region. In 2007 The Washington Post reported on a number of Chinese Internet treatment programs in Beijing. They noted:

" *Sun Jiting spends his days locked behind metal bars in this military-run installation, put there by his parents. The 17-year-old high school student is not allowed to communicate with friends back home, and his only companions are psychologists, nurses and other patients. Each morning at 6:30, he is jolted awake by a soldier in fatigues shouting, "This is for your own good!"*

Sun's offense: Internet addiction.

Alarmed by a survey that found that nearly 14 percent of teens in China are vulnerable to becoming addicted to the Internet, the Chinese government has launched a nationwide campaign to stamp out what the Communist Youth League calls "a grave social problem" that threatens the nation.

Now the country is turning its attention to fighting another, supposed addiction -- one that has been blamed in the state-run media for a murder over virtual property earned in an online game, for a string of suicides and for the failure of youths in their studies.

The Chinese government in recent months has joined South Korea, Thailand and Vietnam in taking measures to try to limit the time teens spend online. It has passed regulations banning youths from Internet cafes and has implemented control programs that kick teens off networked games after five hours.

But no country has gone quite as far as China in embracing the theory and mounting a public crusade against Internet addiction. To skeptics, the campaign dovetails a bit too nicely with China's broader effort to control what its citizens can see on the Internet. The Communist government runs a massive program that limits Web access, censors sites and seeks to control online political dissent.

The clinic in Daxing, a suburb of Beijing, the capital, is the oldest and largest, with 60 patients on a normal day and as many as 280 during peak periods. Few of the patients, who range in age from 12 to 24, are here willingly. Most have been forced to come by their parents, who are paying upward of $1,300 a month -- about 10 times the average salary in China -- for the treatment."

Let's look at the four principles that underlie the treatment of any addiction. These are:

1. Acknowledge and recognize that the addiction is a problem

2. Control and/or cease the addictive activity or behavior

3. Replace the activity or behavior with a more healthy alternative

4. Assist other family members or friends who have been affected by the addiction

1. Recognition

Most addicts use projection ("It's everyone else's fault") and denial ("I don't do it anyway – it's not a problem") as psychological defense mechanisms.... whether their addiction is smoking, alcohol or sex. To get past this and get a picture of the extent of their addiction the addict is asked to keep an objective diary of their Internet behavior. Their partner (who is inevitably angrier and more truthful) may also be interviewed and asked to help in this process.

I have devised a simple questionnaire to detect tele-addiction based on one designed and used world wide to identify alcohol addiction. You can slip these questions into normal conversation with someone you suspect is tele-addicted to identify their level of addiction. I have named this the **RAGE** test for tele-addiction.

Have you unsuccessfully tried to **R**educe your use of the Internet?

Has anyone been **A**ngry with you because of the amount of time you use the Internet?

Have you felt **G**uilty at the amount of time you use the Internet?

Have you **E**scaped from social activity to use the Internet at inappropriate times?

This test requires further scientific validation but, if one draws on the equivalent alcohol addiction test results, people scoring 3 out of 4 would have about a 60 - 70% chance of becoming tele-addicts at some stage in their lives, while those who score 4 out of 4 would have an 85 - 90% chance. Try it yourself and see what you think!

2. Control or cessation

Most addictions are best treated by controlling the behavior and only in exceptional circumstances, where considerable damage is being caused, must people stop the behavior altogether. Examples of this are alcohol and drug abuse. Tele-addicts should try to modify their behavior by restricting their access voluntarily. If this doesn't work, pull out the power plug! Concentrate on other activities for a while then try again at a later stage to reintegrate online activities into your lifestyle.

One patient I recall only managed to reduce his Internet activity when he was made to pay a fine of $5 an hour to the charity of his choice once he went above an agreed one hour per day of online activity! He rapidly learned that he couldn't afford to keep up this activity. The importance of money as a motivator and driver of human behavior should never be under estimated!

Controlling the behavior runs into problems when people "fall in love" with their computer! Dr John Suler calls the phenomenon a *"transference reaction to computers."* Transference, where the patient transfers patterns of thinking and feelings from past relationships to current relationships, is common in online relationships. But transference to a computer! It's true though…. the number of people who give their computers a name and personality is extremely common! I hope this won't be your reaction to your computer failing:

"Lisa's crashed again – she doesn't like wet weather – her hard drive just can't take it. I've got to get her repaired quickly so she can feel OK again. I feel so guilty if I don't look after her properly. It's typical that this should happen now just when I had her hooked up with a really good printer."

Computers can be loved children, as in Lisa's case, powerful parents, erotic partners, good listeners, uncritical friends or can even become part of one's own identity. These computer relationships are often a substitute for unfulfilled needs and, whilst not inherently harmful, they certainly can become so if they become unrealistic, excessive or too intrusive. If people are receiving e- therapy from one of the many counselors on the Internet, transference reactions to the therapist and to the computer may need to be explored and acknowledged as part of the therapeutic process.

2. Behavior replacement

If online time is being reduced then it's important to find fulfilling activities to replace the often enormous amount of time that was previously spent online. The best approach is to look back at what you used to do before you discovered online activities, and what interests you lost as a consequence of your tele-addiction. Some people will want to take up these interests again while others will move in different directions. Much online activity takes place late at night, and it is always worth finding out why the computer is preferred to bed! Stories abound of people in unsatisfactory relationships using online activity as a substitute for these relationships. Others use the computer to develop relationships with new partners.

Esther Gwinnell, in her fascinating book, "Online Seductions" gives many examples of people falling in love with strangers on the Internet. One of the best examples is a letter from "Estherg" to "RainGoddess." Estherg certainly sounds as if she is in love and is spending huge amounts of time on the net-relationship. Attempting to get her to restrict her online activity would presumably be very difficult!

I have fallen in love with a man I met on the Internet – at least, I think it's love. Can it be real love? I've never met him, but we exchange 20 emails a day and spend hours on the phone. I've seen his photograph, and he really turns me on. Frankly my heart just skips a beat when I see his name in my email list. He seems to have everything I want in a man, and I think I love him. But it scares me – how can this be real love? Over the computer? Never having met? Do you think someone can fall in love like this?

One can only imagine how much time it takes to exchange 20 emails per day.

3. Helping the addict's family

Anger. Jealousy. Envy. Exasperation. Fury. Suspicion. Resentment. Mistrust. Loss. Hopelessness.

These are the sorts of emotions commonly reported by the partners or family of tele-addicts. Mostly what they want is the return of a loved one but they also have many issues to work through, not least being the changes they have to make to their own lives once the tele-addict returns to their relationships and has more time for others. How will they cope with this? How has their own life changed to cope with the tele-addiction and do they really want it to go back to how it used to be? If not, what changes do they need to make to make sure the future is satisfying for themselves and their "recovered" partners?

Unfortunately all the advice in the world may not be enough if either the computer, or the online activity, has become part of an individual's identity and reason for being. An anonymous college student put it this way during a chat group:

"It's what I am. Everyone knows me as a computer nerd, and I'm proud of it. It's the only thing I've ever been really good at. I love my computer. Lots of people come to me for advice and it makes me feel really good to be able to help them. Why even the girls who used to ignore me now ask me to help them. It's really important for me to keep my website up to date – everyone thinks it's so cool."
So be careful!
In summary:

- There is a downside to the Internet, and a number of potential risks for patients

- Telephobia exists, despite the Information Age, and we fall into three differing groups in regard to our ability to adopt technology, "eager adopters", "hesitant prove-its" and "resisters".

- The information technology industry is very much a male preserve, and needs to be feminized and made greener

- Excessive use of the Internet is commonly called "Internet addiction" and is associated with "cyberchondria". These are probably not specific identifiable disorders, and are certainly preventable

9

What Does The Future Hold?

The way most doctors and health care professionals do their jobs has hardly changed over the past thirty to forty years. Contrast this with the enormous changes in, say, transport, manufacturing and telecommunications!

But hang on to your stethoscopes! Despite the fact that some doctors still have their heads buried firmly in the sand, the winds of change are blowing and most doctors are using electronic communication technologies, if not enthusiastically, then at least regularly. The combination of technological change, the demands of business and the rise of consumerism are causing radical changes in the way healthcare is practiced around the world. EHealth is poised to revolutionize health practices. The changes will be the 21st century's equivalent of the public health initiatives of sanitation and nutrition which revolutionized health care in the twentieth century. Integration of online technologies will see doctors and patients working together on electronic health records with patients having much more say in their treatments. The development of widely available broadband networks and video mail will bring eHealth into everyone's home. People will be treated in 'virtual hospitals' by global clinicians. Patients and doctors will work collaboratively on the internet as parters with the agreed mutual objective of health improvement. As Dr Rick Satava MD, who has worked with the NASA medical space program for some years has said, "the future isn't what it used to be."

A study by Mercedes Benz shows 12 year olds drive cars better using paddles, as are used in Nintendo games, than adults using steering wheels. As a result the day might not be far off when cars are produced with paddles for steering and the steering wheel is but an optional extra! Look at how fast the average 15 year old can send messages on their phone – gone are the days when a telephone was just an audio device. I use these examples because the way we interact with communication systems is radically changing the way we behave and think in ways that are impossible to predict. And the computer literate children of today - the millenials and succeeding generations - will drive these changes. How many doctors want to interact with patients using instant messaging? Not many today, but the doctors of the millennial generation will probably think nothing of this approach.

Nobody can say with any certainty where or how far the information revolution will take us - not even the computer and information experts! Five years ago they thought they knew but huge advances in information technology have taken them by surprise. Unable to anticipate the changes, the experts are now finally asking the users what they want. This means that, in the health arena, patients and clinicians need to make their demands clear. This is the information age, and it is a far cry from the industrial age of the last century.

In centuries past, land, capital and people have been seen as the economic cornerstones of our society. To these add; "knowledge". The storing of, and passing on, of knowledge from one generation to the next has impacted mightily on the development of the world. Look at the Bible - written two thousand years ago but still the most widely read book in the world. Every day all over the globe its teachings continue to influence people.

Knowledge has never been as important - and as accessible - as it is today. We can describe the changes that started in the late twentieth century as "evolutionary, revolutionary and devolutionary".

EVOLUTION

The evolutionary processes are the new tools, the hardware and software of the computer industries; and changed business processes. In particular we need to substantially redesign many of the traditional processes used to practice medicine so that we can take advantage of the new available multimedia technologies.

Technology, and in particular, Internet technology, is transforming the academic medical landscape. A large number of institutions are moving to digital-only radiography and full electronic medical records. I no longer write any notes on paper – all my clinical work is electronically recorded. House staff now come to rounds armed with a vast array of reference information stored in hand-held personal digital assistants (PDAs). The iPod is a platform for lectures as "podcasts" and "vodcasts" and the feasibility of using an iPod as a mobile x-ray image viewer has been recently demonstrated. Continuing education is also increasingly available through the Internet. The digital revolution has greatly altered how academic health systems pursue education, research, and clinical care.

REVOLUTION

The revolutionary changes are easier access to information and knowledge leading to fringe companies or activities replacing traditional centralized organizations. Many small Internet companies created by young, adventurous people have sprung up overnight and challenged the multi-nationals. The equivalent in health care will be the really good online doctor who might live in, for instance, Montreal, Canada, but who, because of his globally recognized, skills, knowledge, empathy and expertise, attracts patients from all over the world. Many of his patients would have previously gone to local academic centers which will now have to compete on a much more level playing field.

One of the most fundamental transformations is occurring in the area of healthcare delivery. The provision of clinical care is changing rapidly as eHealth technologies become increasingly used and accepted, with a move away from episodic care to concentrating on continuity of care, especially for patients with chronic disease who will create the greatest disease burden in the future. Care is gradually moving away from a focus on the service provider to that of the informed patient and from an individual approach to treatment to a team approach. Increasingly, less focus is placed on treating the illness and more is placed on wellness promotion and illness prevention: the model of the"Information Age care" first described by Dr Tom Ferguson MD. To move to this future of information age healthcare, the availability and use of information must be strengthened to facilitate changes in health service delivery, and a much greater focus must be placed on developing and refining the information technology infrastructure.

A recent report from California headed by Barb Johnston, CEO of the Medical Board of California has summarized this revolution:

"The Digital Age has made access to high-speed broadband services as necessary as telephone service has been for decades. High-speed telecommunications services are now a basic communication tool for education and health, banking, for access to government services, for work-related and marketing activities as well as for leisure activities, games, entertainment and even news."

DEVOLUTION

The devolutionary changes will see organizations becoming more localized and less hierarchical. The world of healthcare will be flatter than it is now. It is only in the last 150 years we have built hospitals - monolithic, hierarchical institutions with complicated administrative processes that are not only threatening to, but can be quite dangerous for patients - evidenced by the number of patients who contract hospital acquired infections or "iatrogenic" – doctor caused – diseases. Over the next fifty or so years many large hospitals, as we know them, will disappear, leaving only a few centers of expertise staffed by super-specialist doctors and other health professionals. Right now we know many thousands of people each year die as a result of medical mistakes in our hospitals, but this should be reduced once we have better information systems that are easily available to all of us. Healthcare will have become a distributed enterprise. We will be able to concentrate our scarce health resources on wellness promotion, instead of just the treatment of illness. There will be more resources available to undertake the mass immunization campaigns that we need around the world and which have in recent times been promoted by the Gates Foundation.

Distributed academic networks of likeminded researchers and clinicians are starting to emerge around the world, and they will not necessarily be based in academic centers. Instead those involved will be in their homes, their businesses or their medical facilities, in any country in the world, in rural and metropolitan areas. They will use grid technologies, multiple computers linked together sharing memory and processing capacity on a daily basis, linked to sophisticated sensors. They will even be potentially controlling software with their minds without the need to lift a finger to control a keyboard, or whatever the interfaces of the future will be. These networks will consist of collaboration of providers, patients, researchers, business people and many others, and they will:

- Empower consumers and clinicians in day-to-day healthcare delivery by improving access to evidence-based information at the point of care;

- Facilitate the delivery of a wider range of health services, particularly to primary and community care;

- Provide accurate data to support research and clinical policy and governance arrangements; and

- Ensure a sustainable, secure, reliable electronic environment, underpinned by strong, policy-driven privacy protection.

Our health system has to meet the challenges contained in the recent crucially important report from the Committee on Quality Healthcare in America published by the Institute of Medicine. This influential report notes that "information technology must play a central role in the redesign of the healthcare system" and suggests that the US needs a renewed national commitment to build an information infrastructure to support healthcare delivery. In addition,*" that commitment should lead to the elimination of most hand written clinical data by the end of the decade."* For this change to occur, the health system has to think seriously about its basic infrastructure requirements, and in the next century, these will increasingly involve close collaboration with telecommunication providers.

NOT ONLY IS THE WORLD CHANGING; IT'S SHRINKING

Our world has changed in the last ten years. The reason we are able to access each other as described in this book is primarily the result of two technologies, fiber optic cabling and satellites. Already millions of kilometers of fiber optic cable connect cities and countries around the world. Cable is now often routinely laid alongside new railway tracks and major roads as part of the infrastructure installed now for use in years to come. In California this "dark fiber", as it is called because it is not yet being used, or lit up, is extraordinarily extensive with the state rail system, Caltrans, being one of the largest owners. Many intercontinental data links are installed. These include massively powerful fiber optic cable weaving from Germany through the Mediterranean, across Southeast Asia and on to Japan and Korea. And while the slow part of the Internet is still the switches that direct data in different directions around the world – the routers - these too are being speeded up using light and laser technologies so that the switches of today are able to handle the equivalent of the entire volume of data carried by the Internet of just ten years ago!

At the same time much improved interactive satellites are being launched – literally in their thousands. Acting like mobile phone towers, or repeaters, they provide worldwide coverage. As the bandwidth or "pipes" broaden, real time interactive video will be increasingly be available all over the world, not just in developed countries as is mainly the case at present. We can all already talk and look at mom, dad, our friends or our doctor on our home monitor anytime we want if you use one of the many Internet video communication systems. And our monitor may be the TV or the computer, on the desk, in the kitchen or perhaps hanging on the wall like a picture! Or you can use the TV to show the latest videos on YouTube via Apple TV. And if you are out and about you can use your phone to see and speak to people using WiFi or cellular technologies available all across the city, or using your inhome wireless network.

The two "pipelines" complement each other. Fiber cables enable information and data to pass very quickly from one point to another: satellites provide total coverage. The world is being quietly wrapped in a cocoon of communications that will bring healthcare ubiquitously to your home.

OPEN-SOURCE COMPUTER APPLICATIONS

This is unfortunately another example of a jargon terminology that describes something that many people poorly understand, but which is important. What are "open source" approaches and methodologies? "Open source" when applied to computer programs means that the source code for an application is available for anyone to review, critique, modify, and redistribute to others. Although access to the source code for modifications and redistribution is important, the transparency and peer review of the open source process is what promotes high quality and reliability in the software. It is free for anyone to modify or change, and allows groups of computer programmers all over the world to work on a single application simultaneously – watching whatever the others are doing, and helping them improve the software. The World Wide Web and the Linux operating system are two examples of wildly successful open source products that have dramatically changed our lives. In the U.S, undoubtedly the most substantial open-source approach to electronic records, among several, has been the Department of Veterans Affairs implementation of "VistA" that started in the 1980's. VistA Lite, downloadable from the Internet, is designed for small medical practices and for non-Veterans Affairs physicians and is in continuing development by a number of developer groups while OpenVistA is another open source derivation of the VistA clinical information system. VistA is used by several healthcare systems outside of the veteran's administration, and at least 56 hospitals in Mexico, with a nation-wide Mexican implementation planned to cover approximately 40 million people.

So what would be the advantages of introducing open-source EHRs widely into the US health environment? Any open-source software initiatives to develop EHRs would draw on the same ethos of peer-review and open discovery that drives much of the research component of the health industry, but at much less expense than current clinical systems. Open-source EHRs would potentially lead to fewer software bugs, lower product costs, continuous improvement, and more custom applications. In the future, patients could access EHRs for health education, to communicate with their healthcare providers, and to add information to their health record. Open-source software technologies could also have important relevance in the area of shareable web-services, connecting directly to your web portal, and other software modules (record locater services, identity services, medication reconciliation services) that could be in an open-source, public library for use by everyone.

I believe we will eventually establish an open-source electronic medical records software effort across the whole healthcare industry, and that this will make cheap electronic records available to us all, and will break the monopoly held by the electronic record companies. This could happen through a series of partnerships between governments, health care organizations, academia, and the private sector with a clear focus on re-aligning the present funding disincentives in healthcare and on improving patient safety and the overall quality of patient care. And this will be a much better long term option as a personal health record than the proprietary records currently being developed by companies like Google and Microsoft. This effort is still some years away, but watch out for it.

DISTRIBUTED EDUCATION

Academic centers and the functions of schools of medicine will be linked with global broadband networks in several ways. Education at medical school will be different in the future, as the schools themselves increasingly become distributed virtual academic environments, available wherever or whenever students need them. Teaching and supervision may be done by specialists from afar who have particular skills or expertise and who are linked to these distributed academic networks. This linking is already happening in some commercial university programs where individual professors, mainly in areas such as business and economics, have become educational "superstars."

The future may bring students who will enroll in a school for basic, hands-on training but who will also enlist in remote lectures for a particular course. Teachers could be sought to "headline" programs and to attract students, in the same way that sports teams hire particular individuals with special talents to ensure success, both on the field and in promoting the brand. The distributed virtual environments of the future could transmit these teachers easily into pre-arranged courses, programs, institutions, and countries, anytime and anywhere. Health education programs may, as a consequence, become more flexible and could become available anywhere. General education companies are already developing specialized courses featuring "star" educators for commercial distribution, and this will undoubtedly happen in the healthcare area. Whether these courses will be distributed by TV, video on the Internet or on CD's will be a matter of individual choice and preference. Look at the example of many websites that now offer educational materials in video format, often loaded up to YouTube as well, including the Web Video Editorials and other multimedia offerings from The Medscape Journal of Medicine (www.medscape.com).

WHAT IS INTERNET 2?

In brief it is the next generation of the Internet, built and managed primarily by research universities, and focused on research and education, and the requirements of the international research community. Its mission is to ensure that researchers have access to the most advanced networking capabilities required for the next generation of what is now called "cyberinfrastructure-enabled, collaborative discovery". What this means is that Internet2 is the research road on which other applications drive. President Clinton described the effort in his 1997 State of the Union Address:

"We must build the second generation of the Internet so that our leading universities and national laboratories can communicate one thousand times faster than today. But we cannot stop there. As the Internet becomes our new home and town square, a computer in every home – a teacher of all subjects, a connection to all cultures, this will no longer be a dream but a necessity."

The Internet 2 consortium is made up of people from most major American universities and many commercial partners. It has two main goals:

- "To design, operate and continually enhance the world's leading research and education network

- To provide researchers and scholars with the tools and support they need to envision and execute the next generation of transformational cyberinfrastructure-enabled discovery"

The Internet2 website at www.Internet2.edu describes a compelling vision of their future directions. They imagine a network that:

- "Allows researchers to collaborate in real time using high-definition audio and video that's as good as being there

- Supports collaborative use of a wide range of tools including globally distributed environmental sensor networks, advanced telescopes on remote mountaintops, distributed databases, digitally rich performance environments and immersive virtual reality

- Reaches not only around the world but into health and education institutions in every corner of our nation."

Internet2 has already had major benefits.

Internet2 is radically changing the way we work, play and do business! It is particularly exciting for health. We are able to develop fully digitalized libraries which include not just text but comprehensive video and audio collections. We can build collaborative virtual research laboratories enabling "tele-immersion" - the ability to move inside space, inside the human body and into virtual reality situations, where several people can share space at the same time. Surgeons and students are able to literally immerse themselves inside a three dimensional virtual middle ear, allowing the surgeons to teach the anatomy, pathology and surgery of the ear to their students inside that organ!

Combine the communications revolution with the genetic discoveries associated with the largest international scientific research project in the history of the world, the Human Genome Project, where our genes are being explored and typed, and the prospects for future health care are amazing and exciting. The field of genomics, where we use our genetic knowledge to prevent and treat illness, will combine with the fields of nanotechnology and robotics, where miniaturized physiological and other man made devices are being programmed to literally operate on us from inside our bodies. And these exciting advances will be supported by the communications revolution that well underway.

EHEALTHCARE FOR THE NEW MILLENNIUM

Institutions and paper medical records will go out the window. The patient will come first. Wellness will be promoted, patients will receive continuous care in the community in an active partnership with their doctors. Computerized records owned by patients and shared with their doctors will tie everything together. Paperless hospitals will be common. In time the computer, television, telephone, telemedicine systems and other technologies will be integrated into a single interactive communications technology product or platform. No one has thought of a good name for this yet although the iPod probably comes closest of all the available current technologies. Health care professionals will use it to access patient records, videoconference with colleagues and patients, link to library, financial and administrative programs and systems and attend to all their personal requirements too.

Not everyone will have this interactive device at home but, just as we have commercial 'Internet cafes' and numerous "hot spots" now, so I believe public "telecenters" will spring up where people will be able to access their records or use other parts of the Internet with extraordinary speed. This will be especially important in the underdeveloped nations where the communications revolution will allow much more rapid social and economic development than would otherwise have been possible.

Major teaching hospitals will not escape the winds of change. As broadband networks effectively spread knowledge to every corner of the globe there'll be less need for teaching hospitals in every city. Instead, I suspect, teaching hospitals or tertiary field centers, servicing whole states or countries, will emerge to provide super-specialist procedures not available in community-based centers.

These tertiary centers will service not only countries but international time zones. Up until now we have got on pretty well by carving earth up into continents and countries. However, the world of the future is more likely to be divided into three different time zones because, despite all our accumulated knowledge, we still haven't found a way around the need for human beings to sleep! It is unlikely clinicians in a major tertiary hospital in, for instance, New York, will want to service patients in India who are in an almost opposite time zone. These three time zones are likely to comprise, firstly, North and South America, secondly, Europe, Western Russia, India and Africa, and thirdly, Eastern Russia, Asia and Australasia.

It will be interesting to see if a major teaching hospital in Rio de Janeiro is able to compete with an equivalent institution in Washington, DC, to provide services to patients in Mexico!

Present day health businesses are mostly a hotch potch of small cottage industries, powerful autocratic empires or protected, poorly defined hierarchies that not even the doctors who work within them can understand. Just as businesses have become more flexible, and major companies have become enterprises, partnering with each other in different ways at different points in time depending on their needs, so will healthcare groups become enterprises. This added flexibility will provide more choice for patients as these health enterprises expand and contract in response to clinical demands and needs, rather than through historical forces.

This approach will demand significant efficiencies, and changes, in the training and practice of all health professionals, especially doctors. Medical schools, and other health care education institutions, will have to entirely change their teaching curricula. Being the Dean of a medical school, typically a conservative profession, will be very difficult over the next 20 years.

While clinicians have embraced some communication technologies such as telephones, mobiles, faxes, pagers, tape recorders and TV's, sadly, computers are only just now being put to good clinical use, although not yet routinely for communicating with patients. Instead they are mostly used by doctors for accounting and scheduling purposes, as well as for information searching and retrieval. But this is all changing.

Shopping Around

As the brave new world emerges there is no reason why you shouldn't "visit" a surgeon, nutritionist, physician or nurse – all based in different areas around your country or global timezone. Your insurance plan is soon likely to be your major barrier. Multidisciplinary health care teams, preferably co-ordinated by your local primary care face to face doctor are inevitable. This will mean, over time, a complete re-engineering of health systems both inside countries, and globally. In the US this will cause major difficulties because of the entrenched positions by all of those with a stake in the old inefficient paper driven system - the many for-profit driven health institutions. Equally entrenched are the lawyers who put up the cost of medicine so dramatically by constantly facilitating legal suits against doctors, who defensively respond by over ordering tests and investigations to protect themselves, at your, the patients, cost.

Fortunately the arrival of ubiquitously available broadband networks will leave these health vultures high and dry in their well-feathered nests. Whether they like it or not Internet 2 and related networks will put video eHealth activities on everyone's desktop wherever they may be in the world. It will be fascinating to see how this affects the US healthcare industry. Will we see true international competition in health? Physicians in Australia typically charge between US$100 and US$150 an hour. In the United States rates are usually at least double. Market forces are likely to dictate. Some patients will choose cheaper treatment by equally qualified overseas doctors. As a potential consumer, I personally have no problem seeking an opinion from a world expert situated, say, in London, New York or Toronto. If they also happen to be cheaper than my local physician, I am doubly blessed!

Obviously, issues of policy, legality and medical registration will need to be sorted out around the world, as at the moment, most doctors and other health professionals are only registered within their own countries. But this will happen. Consumers will demand that it happens.

Patient Power

We are not only living in the age of information technology, it is also the age of consumerism. For many reasons health has probably been one area least affected by the rise of consumerism - but this is about to change. Patients must become more involved in the debate on the future of eHealth and health care delivery? They are the pivotal points in a system that has, for so long, focused mainly on the needs of clinicians. Some have proposed an international "patient's bill of rights" - a great idea incorporating a global perspective. After all, why shouldn't an online patient in Russia have the same rights as one in Baltimore?

Dr Tom Ferguson, was very critical of the type of health information provided by doctors to patients - he called it "shovelware." Shovelware consists of the typical patient information pamphlets that you see in your doctor's office - often produced by drug companies, and offering generic, and very general, information. Ferguson researched the type of information patients want, working with a very, in his words, a "net-savvy" group of health consumers. The results were commonsense. Patients want replies to their specific questions, individualized information presented interactively, the results of health searches that are specific to their problem and information about the best sites for their problem. The emergence of better health information has certainly changed the way patients understand their diseases and will greatly assist the majority of patients in their quest for good treatment. What examples of patient power!

THE WIDER BENEFITS FOR ALL OF US

The tangible benefits of eHealth are already obvious. The pediatric telemedicine program run by Dr Jim Marcin at my own medical center, UC Davis, is an example that has been highlighted by Governor Arnold Swarzenegger who undertook his own first distance consultation in 2006. Here children in intensive care units or emergency rooms around Northern California are linked by videoconferencing to Dr Marcin and his colleagues for urgent assessments, and if they are transferred to UC Davis, sometimes after a rapid helicopter flight, they can then be linked back from to their parents in their rural home community, also by video. In this case telemedicine is being used to provide emotional, educational and medical support to families of hospitalized children, as well as for urgent medical assessments.

In future families will be able to make video visits to loved ones in hospital when it is not convenient to physically visit, saving time and energy. Not only will this be good for maintaining their relationships, but think of the gas that will be saved through less travel. After all, one gallon of gas leads to twenty pounds of polluting carbon emissions, so using these systems has the potential to help us reduce environmental damage significantly. And video visits will not only be confined to hospitals - whenever we are away from home on work, holiday or even in prison we will be able to keep in touch by video! The use of video on broadband networks is going to change our lives more than we can possibly imagine as we discover more and more applications for it. It really will be a case of "seeing is believing."

CHANGING THE WAY DOCTORS WORK

Doctors are starting to redesign the way they work to link better with patients and to use the newly available multi-media technologies. This is a really important process that will undoubtedly accelerate over the next 20 years, and which will help bring out the vision of medical care that is being presented in this book. I believe it is time to substantially redesign many of the traditional processes we use to practice medicine.

As we do this, doctors need to follow two core principles. The first is the complementarity principle - computers do well, what humans do badly, and vice versa. Computers never forget, and are great at scheduling, remembering and reminding, but humans are much better at data analysis and decision making. The second principle is the importance of redesigning business processes before building new software environments – that one should not design new software to support an old inefficient business process. This has unfortunately happened in many areas of the health community in the past, and only now are doctors starting to realize that they should be professionally analyzing their workflows, and making changes to their "production" to be more effective. This is something that Toyota did many years ago. While many doctors don't like to admit it, there are a lot of similarities between the car production line, and the practice of medicine. And doctors can learn from engineers in this area.

We will increasingly think differently, for example, about the doctor-patient consultation as discussed earlier in this book. It can be described as consisting of three information processes – data capture (history and examination), data analysis (diagnosis), and business planning (treatment). Using the principles mentioned previously we can now start to identify which components are best undertaken by the various humans involved, and which are best undertaken automatically or in a technology driven manner. We can literally break down the historically developed medical practice process and build it again from scratch – just as if we were designing a new factory to build Toyotas.

I am a strong believer in store and forward, or asynchronous medicine. All this means is that in many instances I am confident it is possible for a doctor to give an opinion about a patient without seeing them in person, or in real time. After all, when was the last time you met a radiologist or a pathologist. These specialists have been working in this way for years. Other doctors or technicians take x-rays, or provide specimens, and describe the clinical history, and the radiologist or pathologist then takes all that data, examines it, and gives an opinion that can be used by the patients treating doctor. This sort of approach is increasingly being used in cardiology (with ultrasounds and EKG's) dermatology (pictures of the skin lesions) and ophthalmology (retinal photographs) to provide specialist opinions to primary providers. It works, and it is more rapid and easily undertaken for all involved, especially for the patient, who no longer has to travel and take time off work to see a specialist.

If it works in those specialties, why shouldn't it work in specialties like psychiatry or neurology, where it is easy enough to take video clips of patient interviews as the core data source, combined with background information, and where other medical information, such as blood tests and x-rays can be sent as well. And why shouldn't it be possible to do these consultations across a number of different languages, by having written translations on screen added to the videos by professional interpreters so that, for instance, Spanish speaking patients may be interviewed in their native language, but be assessed by English speaking psychiatrists observing clips of their interviews translated on screen as in the movies, 24 hours later.

I am testing exactly this notion - of store and forward cross language telepsychiatry consultations, right now. I and my team are working with rural primary care providers in central California. We upload psychiatric clinical datasets and short patient video clips in English or Spanish to our secure website. These datasets are examined by English or Spanish speaking psychiatrists who create and upload diagnostic assessments and treatment plans, translated as required. The psychiatrist's opinions are then instantly available for the primary care providers in the language of their choice. Doesn't this make sense? It obviates the need for patients and specialists to travel and physically meet. It makes specialists accessible to patients living in isolated areas who would not normally be able to have such access. It means that the extra complication of arranging a physical interpreter for a consultation is no longer necessary. And if I, as the store and forward consultant, want a physical examination performed, then all I have to do is ask the primary provider to do it, on video if necessary, and send me the results.

Patients need to encourage doctors to think of ways of redesigning their practice processes to make better use of available multimedia technologies so that they can continue to provide better and more available care. I am sure this will happen, especially as more of the "millennial" generation start receiving care. They will demand that doctors use these technologies, and increasingly change their ways.

TEACHING OUR CHILDREN WELL

Children, more than any other group, have embraced online technology with a passion and we shouldn't pass up this golden opportunity to instill healthy lifestyle habits. By the time they turn twelve most children have already acquired lifelong behaviors. After this, many "switch off" learning new life skills of a preventive nature. Fortunately their brains "switch on" again when they reach about twenty-five but by that time a proportion will have already suffered many life traumas – such as drug and alcohol abuse, relationship break ups and instability, or unwanted pregnancies at a time in their life that should be exciting and fun.

Children in western countries are quite at home on computers but sadly most computer games are "mindless" and teach them little more than how to manipulate a joystick or keyboard. What we must do is develop challenging and exciting computer games and online programs which deliver effective health care and lifestyle messages. We know that even very young children are highly receptive to educational messages. Marketing is crucial and can be seen in the success of companies like McDonalds and Coca-Cola who, through aggressive education and marketing campaigns, have managed to become part of our children's culture causing lifelong behavioral and psychological dependence on, and interest in, "junk food"!

We need to move beyond the "quit smoking" campaigns to online education campaigns which prevent people from taking up smoking in the first place. We need to develop "child friendly" educational multi-media games for primary school children that will be fun to play but which also carry clear preventive health messages. Programs that can be used as part of the school health curriculum, facilitated by teachers, and which involve families and communities, not just children, as health interventions, not just health education. Perhaps one title might be "Doom defies Dope"! A great title to use to explore the importance of power in relationships and to teach children and families about ways of avoiding abuse and violence. The use of online technologies to improve the health prospects of the next generation is an exciting prospect and within our grasp – and the younger generations have the skills and attitudes to use them well.

So what principles should be used to build these online education environments?

There are a number of basic principles of adult learning that can be used online and which are very different from either traditional textbook or classroom-based education. We need to use these principles to teach more intelligently, and the online world is ideally suited for them. Adult learning emphasizes the importance of active rather than passive learning. This approach ensures that learners are interactively involved with their educational materials and resources, are encouraged to ask questions, make comments, and contribute examples from their own experience throughout their learning program. Often learners are given specific sets of assessment tasks to perform during their learning activity as continuous assessment that is for their eyes only, and is not part of the final, assessment that they undertake. Very often active learning is problem-based or case-based. Here a short educational trigger from a relevant problem is given to the student, or group of students, who then work out learning objectives, and then content requirements, that are needed to solve the problem, and they do it as a group, potentially from their computers anywhere in the world. Problem-based learning, which is strongly focused on decision making capacities and reasoning processes, is ideal for the healthcare field, and this strategy is now being employed by quite a number of medical schools around the world, representing a substantial move away from traditional classroom and laboratory-based curricula. Students typically find problem-based learning to be more relevant, and to be more closely linked to their real world clinical learning experiences.

Equally important, in terms of adult learning approaches and principles, are what are increasingly being called "just-in-time" learning experiences. This is essentially "on the job" learning, whereby the learner is provided with educational information literally at the time they need it. For example, a resident in a busy clinic is able to use an online decision support tool to access pharmaceutical information to guide their prescribing, or can quickly find a clinical guideline on which to base their treatment plan. Such educational opportunities are increasingly being recognized as being an important component of many graduate programs in particular.

The final major component of adult learning is the capacity of the learner to access and integrate multiple sources of information, and to be able to evaluate the quality of those sources so they can form a judgment as to what is useful information for them to use at any particular time. Traditional learners in the pre-Internet world used to depend on the reputations of textbooks and papers by learned authors published by authoritative groups, but in the Internet world it is much more difficult to be confident of the reliability and validity of much of the information that appears on easily available generic search engines such as Google.

JUST IN TIME LEARNING

"Just in time" learning is the key issue from a student perspective. It is well known that most students now own two core electronic appliances, the cellular telephone and an iPod, blackberry or equivalent instrument. Our present generation of students is used to multi-tasking, to receiving music downloads, instant messaging, and using phones as ubiquitous instruments for Internet access and photography in addition to communication. Podcasting allows students to download files directly to their iPods or computers, and then to listen to the files at their leisure, and is a sure forerunner to Vodcasting, the streaming of video to iPod instruments, which is increasingly appearing via iTunes and YouTube.

A number of other more technically high-powered environments will also be increasingly used for adult learning-based education approaches in the future, the most obvious of which is the use of virtual reality programs, either on the Internet, via headsets, or using specialized 3D rooms, often called "caves". I have been using a multi-user commercial platform (www. secondlife.com) to develop 3D environments on the Internet where learners navigate digital representations of themselves, called "avatars", through a 3D virtual psychiatric ward. This system is designed to help students learn more about the subjective experience of psychosis and, ultimately, to improve care to their patients. Users can literally see and hear hallucinations as a patient might, as they"walk" through the halls of the virtual "hospital". The auditory and visual hallucinations themselves are based on the real lived experiences of a number of patients, which have then been recreated using multimedia techniques. There are clearly a number of other areas in where virtual reality technologies can be applied. There are already avatar virtual therapists in Second Life, with patients logging in as avatars from any number of different sites to meet their therapist online. And there is the potential for treatment of addictions, obesity, anxiety, and pain, and the development of some specific programs for obsessions, phobias, and related fears. This whole area, recently termed "serious games", is full of exciting innovations that increasingly make sense from an educational perspective. Watch this space. You will see much more of this type of education, and therapy, in future.

A Better Understanding of Illness

For doctors to feel at first hand what their patients are going through is literally mind-boggling - but this is another benefit of online technology. The first time I, as a psychiatrist, experienced simulations of auditory hallucinations, a common symptom of schizophrenia, was at the American Psychiatric Association meeting in San Diego in 1997. A pharmaceutical company was demonstrating an audiotape they had developed. Seated in a sound-proof booth, wearing headphones, I was subjected to stereo hallucinations which seemed to come from every direction inside my head. At the same time I was trying to take part in a mock interview. The experience was both eerie and fascinating. It was extremely difficult to concentrate on the interviewer's questions, never mind organize a coherent answer, while being constantly interrupted by unpredictable voices and noises. For the first time in 15 years of practicing psychiatry I had an inkling of what it must be like to be psychotic and hallucinating. I certainly wouldn't have passed the job interview. It was a great learning experience and should be mandatory for anyone working with people suffering from schizophrenia or other forms of psychosis. I can now understand something of what they are experiencing.

We will go much further than this however. I can see a time in maybe ten to twenty years when it will be possible, using information technology and virtual reality techniques, to almost perfectly recreate many medical and psychiatric disorders in cyberspace. A patient with, say, early symptoms of epilepsy, Alzheimer's disease, depression or schizophrenia, perhaps including hallucinations of voices and touches, will join their doctor in a virtual reality "booth". The doctor will be able to recreate the patient's exact symptoms using virtual reality techniques to help in diagnosing and monitoring the disorder. Doctor's won't have to rely just on verbal descriptions of symptoms and our own observations of patients' behavior as we do at present. The forerunners of these booths are already being built and are called "caves" – literally 3 dimensional rooms where you feel like you have entered a new world. The diagnostic possibilities of combining virtual reality approaches to diagnosis, with artificial intelligence programs that continuously learn, and become more accurate in their predictions, as more data is fed to them, and the connectivity and power of Internet 2 are almost limitless.

AFFECTIVE COMPUTING – COMPUTERS HAVE FEELINGS, TOO

Far fetched as it sounds it is already possible for information to be electrically passed along a line of people holding hands with terminals attached to the legs of the person at each end of the line! I know this sounds weird but we all know we transmit electricity and must wear rubber shoes when repairing electrical equipment. It is therefore logical, even if it seems unreal right now, that we could literally be a part of the information system! Dr Andy Lippman from the Massachusetts Institute of Technology Media Laboratory, who describes himself as a "digital futurist" has described this future of "affective computing" - computing with feelings. Others are looking at how to transmit smells, or signals identifying smells, over the Internet – this is perhaps somewhat easier as it is possible to have digital signals transmitted that encode for specific smells, and release them, from one end of a line to another. The term "natural interfacing" is used by scientists who are studying the mechanics of how to allow humans to interact via computers in a way similar to talking to each other – without a need for a keyboard, pad or stylus.

The ultimate goal for these researchers is to design systems that can interact directly with our minds – allowing sounds and ideas to be transmitted straight into our brains, allowing us to merge seamlessly with machines. In this view of the future people will have wearable mini-computers that understand the rhythm, inflection, tone and emphasis of speech, and that can respond in a human sounding manner – very different from the mechanical sounding computer speech we have now.

What could this mean for patients? If you are depressed you may have, in a few years time, a "depression monitor" strapped to your arm. On particularly bad days the monitor could transmit a message to your doctor letting him know to contact you. Perhaps this will finally be the sort of technology that will help prevent suicides. You might also have your heart monitored (by EKG), a temperature monitor, and your brain electrical activity recorded (by EEG). We know that animals can literally smell fear, and maybe one day we will be able to recreate these types of senses. Researchers are already detecting all sorts of disorders and abnormalities in exhaled breath – it is not to far out to suggest that instead of patients having blood tests in future, that they will have breath tests, just as we routinely use to screen for alcohol levels. After all, exhaled cells can be captured and a persons DNA examined within cells that have come from the lining of the lungs, so why should we stick with blood. Breath examination could possibly lead to continuous physiological monitoring tools, with outputs electronically shared in real time via wireless monitors worn in clothes creating a "virtual body local area network" connected to the Internet, and a monitoring service.

Such technology is not in the realms of fantasy. It sounds a bit like the downside of 1984, the cult book by George Orwell, but is a big advance on today's movement or cardiac monitors which are linked to twenty four hour central monitoring services and are voluntarily worn by many elderly folk. If the gauges look abnormal the service rings the patient, or in some instances, sends an ambulance out. Suicidal depression is as much an emergency as heart failure and hopefully in the future it will be monitored just like diabetes, heart disease and asthma. Undoubtedly lives will be saved.

EVERY FACE TELLS A STORY – DISTRIBUTED INTELLIGENCE

Our faces show our emotions. They are the window of our feelings. Clinicians are trained to both consciously and unconsciously pick up diagnostic cues from patients' faces. We know what someone physically looks like when they are depressed but we can't physiologically describe it. We know their brow is furrowed, their mouth drawn, their skin looks dry and pasty and that they are tearful and their face moves slowly. Soon we will be able to mathematically measure and model our facial features by converting a video to digital data. Visual diagnostic tests will also be used to assess strokes, neurological movement disorders, even side-effects of medication. And much more accurately than we can do so at present.

These visual X-rays will be combined with simple facial sensors, such as are already being used by Dr Dave Warner, another futurist.. He believes that we will eventually have multi-media patient records which particularly concentrate on patients' faces. These will give us much more objective information to assist in patient care. And of course patients will be able to use sensors at home to give them more control over their treatment options. Meanwhile Dr Rick Satava, another futuristic guru, talks of a 3-dimensional model of the human body, with multiple MRI scans showing internal physical details, and digitized pictures showing the outside. This is the ultimate visual medical record. Whilst the biochemical aspects of this vision are still some years away, we have excellent scanned 3D internal pictures already available that are routinely used in many areas of surgery.

A SINGLE VISUAL DISPLAY OF YOUR WHOLE MEDICAL RECORD?

Blaise Aguera y Arcas is an architect at Microsoft Live Labs, and the co-creator of Photosynth, an amazing piece of software capable of assembling static photos into a synergy of zoomable, navigatable spaces. This seamless patchwork of images can be viewed via multiple angles and magnifications, allowing you to look around corners or "fly" in for a (much) closer look. Imagine that you are looking at pictures of Google earth – you can zoom in from an enormous height and literally look in your backyard on photos originally taken from space. Well what Blaise has created is software that allows you to put whole collections of photographs, of books, of newspapers, on a single screen, and then have you zoom in and out to all areas of the screen. You can easily find any photo or paragraph where ever you want, without the need for any of the tabs or content lists that we have to use at the moment to move around our small piece of computer real estate – our monitor.

Why is this potentially important in healthcare? Think of your electronic medical record – it is a massively difficult piece of software to navigate – literally hundreds of pages of data, results, x-rays, lab tests, letters and the like. Wouldn't it be so much easier if the whole record of your life, and your health, could literally be laid out in front of you so that you, and your doctor, could navigate around it – could easily zoom from place to place – from consultation note, to x-ray – from lab result to photograph? Suddenly your electronic health record would have come alive – you and your doctor would be able to easily find relevant parts of your record, which would appear almost like a single map, visually searchable. What a difference from the record we use now, and how much easier for everyone to use. What if this was combined with "surface computing", a new technology that literally turns your coffee table into a visualization space where you can move images and pages around, and link them wirelessly to your camera or iPod, shifting data back and forth between the "coffee table" and your devices? You could then literally look at your whole health record on the "kitchen table", or on a shared desk space in your doctor's office. This is a whole new world in comparison to today's computer screens – no longer would you doctor be sitting at his desk typing notes, instead he would be sitting across from you as you both shared your record, perhaps adding and subtracting files from your iPhone, and his blackberry. You would be able to leave the consultation with a fully electronic treatment plan, copies of your most recent x-rays, and perhaps a video of some of your physical signs, such as your infected throat, taken during the examination, all available on whichever wireless device you were carrying that day.

ARE WE CLOSE TO UTOPIA?

Before we get too self congratulatory, hold on! There is no point in being clever enough to invent all these new technologies if we don't use them properly.

Wikipedia defines **techno-utopia** as "*a hypothetical ideal* society, *in which* laws, government, *and* social conditions *are solely operating for the benefit and well-being of all its citizens, set in the near- or far*-future, *when advanced* science and technology *will allow these ideal living standards to exist; for example,* post scarcity, changes in human nature and the human condition, *the* absence of suffering *and even the* end of death.*"

In place of the static perfection of a utopia, others have envisioned an "extropia," an evolving open society allowing individuals and voluntary groupings to form the institutions and social forms they prefer.

We have to be careful not to be "techno-Utopians" - excessively, uncritically acceptance of technologies. People like this don't tend to use new technologies as effectively as they could because they view the technologies as ends in themselves not as tools. It is commonly held that using new technologies uncritically implies bad habits of the mind. Taking television as an example, one could argue that this technology has led us to concentrate on superficial, rapid acquisition of knowledge rather than on deep thinking and careful consideration. Look at all the "newsbites" prepared for TV – and how if you are trained in media skills, you are almost always taught to literally speak in "bites".

On a more positive note Dr Dave Warner has this to say:

"As an information bank the Internet has massively fostered an awareness of human health and the possibilities for its improvement. Medicine on the global information highway is not just going to be reserved for the type of practitioner who comes from a Western medical school and was trained in a hospital. The content will be profoundly diverse. There is no precedent for medicine in cyberspace. Everything from basic vitamin approaches to acupuncture, homoeopathy, psychic healing, past life regression and psychedelic shamanism are flourishing to one degree or another."

And he's optimistic about the future of health online -

"Out of these ideas and with this technology there will emerge a culture of medical Cybernauts committed to creating a world of healthy individuals, families and communities, enhancing the quality of life."

Healthcare on the Internet, in partnership with your doctor, promises huge benefits not only for us all, patients, clinicians and society in general. But in embracing the technology, the human factor must not be forgotten. It is not the cleverness of the technology that is important but how we use it to derive most benefit for us, for our children, and for society. We have to learn to improve, to control, and to effectively use the tools and techniques discussed in this book to improve our health and, in doing this, to enrich the quality of our lives.

In this world there are those who make things happen, those who watch what happens, and those who wonder what happened. Let us make sure that we are in the first group with our doctors.

To summarize future directions and issues:

- "The future isn't what it used to be" as we move to the era of virtual hospitals and global clinicians

- Our health system is gradually changing and becoming electronic and distributed, with less dependency on buildings, and more on communication networks from the patients home to the operating theater

- Research is opening up whole new ways of delivering healthcare, using all our senses, and in a much more personalized manner

- Patients are demanding better and more accessible healthcare, and will obtain it from all around the world in future

- The doctor-patient relationship is changing, and will become increasingly open and driven by empowered patients living in an information rich environment – where the Internet is increasingly influential and important in clinical consultations.

REFERENCES AND FURTHER READING

The following list of references are a combination of those quoted in this book and some others that I believe will be of particular interest to readers who wish to explore some of the issues raised in this book in more depth.

References

Adler, J. (2008). Just the Tree of Us. *Newsweek* (April 14), 42-48.

Ainsworth, M. (n.d.) "Online Therapy." <http:// www.cmhc.com/guide/ cyber.html>

Allen, A., and Grigsby, B. (1998). Consultation Activity in 35 Specialties. Telemedicine Today (October), 18-19.

Allen, A., Cristoferi, A., Campana, S., and Grimaldi, A. (1997). An Italian telephone-mediated home monitoring service: TeSAN Pesonal Emergency Response System & Teleservices. Telemedicine Today (December), 25-33.

Amenta, F., Dauri, A., and Rizzo, N. (1998). Telemedicine and medical care to ships without a doctor on board. *Journal of Telemedicine and Telecare,* 4 (Supp.1), 44-45.

Auerbach, P. S. Physicians and the Environment. *JAMA,* 299(8), 956-958.

Baer, L., Cukor, P., and Jenike, M., et al. (September 1995). Pilot Studies of Telemedicine for Patients with Obsessive-Compulsive Disorder. *American Journal of Psychiatry,* 152(9).

Balas, E. Andrew, Jaffrey, F., and Kuperman, G.J. et al. (July 9, 1997). Electronic Communication with Patients – Evaluation of Distance Medicine Technology. *Journal of the American Medical Association,* 278(2).

Balch, D. C., Warner, D. C., Gustke, S. S. (1999). Medical knowledge on demand. Highlights from the third DMI Conference. *MD Computing,* (March-April) 16(20), 48-50.

Ball, C., et al. (1998). Videoconferencing and the hard of hearing. *Journal of Telemedicine and Telecare,* 4, 57-59.

Ball, C. and Puffett, A. (1998). The assessment of cognitive function in the elderly using videoconferencing. *Journal of Telemedicine and Telecare,* 4 (Supp.1), 36-38.

Bashshur, R. (1997). Clinical Issues in Telemedicine. *Telemedicine Journal,* 3(2).

Bristol, N. (February 10, 2007). US health-care providers go "green." *The Lancet,* 369, 453-4.

Brosnan, M. (1998). Technophobia: The psychological impact of information technology. New York: Routledge.

Cairncross, F. (1997). *The death of distance: How the communications revolution will change our lives.* Boston: Harvard Business School Press.

Coeira, E. (1997). *Guide to Medical Informatics, the Internet and Telemedicine.* New York: Oxford University Press.

De Leo, G. M., Ponder, T., Molet, M., Fato, D., Thalmann and N. Magnenat-Thalmann et al. (2003). A virtual reality system for the training of volunteers involved in health emergency situations. *Cyberpsychol Behav,* 6, 267-74.

Diederich, J., and Yellowlees, P. (n.d.). Ex-ray: Machine learning for the assessment of mental health. Paper presented at the Proceedings of the Conference on Neuro-Computing and Evolving Intelligence, Auckland, New Zealand.

Doolittle, et al. (1998). Hospice care using home-based telemedicine systems. *Journal of Telemedicine and Telecare,* 4(1), 58-9.

Doolittle, G. (1997). A POTS-based tele-hospice project in Missouri. *Telemedicine Today* (August).

Ferguson, T. (October 21, 1998). Digital doctoring – opportunities and challenges in electronic patient-physician communication. *JAMA,* 280(15), 1361-2.

Gamberini, L., P. Cottone, A. Spagnolli, D. Varotto, and G. Mantovani. (2003). Responding to a fire emergency in a virtual environment: Different patterns of action for different situations. *Ergonomics,* 46, 842-58.

Gammon, D., T. Sorlie, S. Bergvik, and T. Sorensen Hoifodt. (1998.) Psychotherapy supervision conducted by videoconferencing: A qualitative study of users' experiences. *Journal of Telemedicine and Telecare,* 4(Supp.1), 33-35.

Gladwell, M. (2005). *Blink.* New York: Time Warner.

Gladwell, M. (2000). *The Tipping Point.* New York: Little, Brown and Company

Gray J., et al. (1998). Telematics in the neonatal ICU and beyond: Improving care, communication and information sharing. *Medinfo,* 9(1), 294-97

Golkaramnay, V., Bauer, S., Haug, S., Wolf, M., and Kordy, H. (2008). The exploration of the effectiveness of group therapy through an Internet chat as aftercare: A controlled naturalistic study. New York: *Psychotherapeutics Research*

Griffiths, L., Blignault, I., and Yellowlees, P. (2006). Telemedicine as a means of delivering cognitive behavior therapy to rural and remote mental health clients. *Journal of Telemedicine and Telecare,* 12(3), 136-40.

Grohol, J. (1999). The insider's guide to mental health Resources Online. New York: Guilford Press.

Groopman, J. (2007). *How Doctors Think.* New York: Houghton Mifflin Books.

Gwinnell, E. (1998). Online Seductions. New York: Kodansha America, Inc.

Hancock, J. (2007). *Digital Deception.* In The Oxford Handbook of Internet Psychology, 289-302. New York: Oxford University Press.

Hilty, D. M., Marks, S. L., Urness, D., Yellowlees, P. M., and Nesbitt, T. (August 2003). Clinical and Educational Applications of Telepsychiatry: A Review. *Canadian Journal of Psychiatry ,* 49(1), 12-23.

Hilty, D. M., Yellowlees, P. M., Cobb, H. C., Neufeld, J. C., and Bourgeois, J. A. (April 2006). The eMental Health Consultation Service: Providing Enhanced Primary Care Mental Health Services through Telemedicine. *Psychosomatics,* 47, 152-157.

Hilty, D., Yellowlees, P., Cobb, H. S., Bourgeois, J. A., Neufeld, J.D., and Nesbitt, T.S. (March-April 2006). Models of telepsychiatric consultation-liaison service to rural primary care. *Psychosomatics,* 47(2), 152-7.

Hilty, D. M., Yellowlees, P. M., Cobb, H., Neufeld, J., Bourgeois, J. A. Use of secure e-mail and telephone: Psychiatric consultations to accelerate rural health service delivery. *Telemed J E Health,* 12(4), 490-5.

Hodges, L. F. et al. Graphics, Visualisation and Usability Centre. College of Computing at Georgia Tech. <http://www.cc.gatech.edu>

Itzhak, B., Weinberger, T., Berkovitch, E., and Reis, S. (1998). Telemedicine in primary care in Israel. *Journal of Telemedicine and Telecare,* 4 (Supp.1), 11-14.

Junnarkar, S. (1997). *Telepsychiatry: Healing Minds Despite Distance.* New York.

Joinson, A., McKenna, K., Postmes, T., and Ulf-Dietrich, R. (2007). *The Oxford Handbook of Internet Psychology.* New York: Oxford University Press.

Kane, B., and Sands, D. Z. (1998.) Guidelines for the Clinical Use of Electronic Mail with Patients. *Journal of the American Medical Informatics Assoc.,* (January/February), 5(1).

Kraut, R., et al. (September 1998). Internet paradox: A social technology that reduces social involvement and psychological well-being? *American Psychologist*, 53(9), 1017-31.

Kushner, D. (2003). *Masters of doom: How two guys created an empire and transformed pop culture.* New York: Random House.

Leamon, M., Miller, M., and Kozol, N. (eds.). (2000). Amphetamine Epidemics. In M. DeClercq, et al. *Emergency Psychiatry in a Changing World, Part XI,* 377-81.

New York: Elsevier Science.

Ledeen, K. S. Build v. Buy: A Decision Paradigm For Information Technology Applications. <http://nevo.com/our-knowledge/whitepapers.asp>

Lesselroth, B. (2008). Clinicians Must Reinvent the Medical Record to Stimulate the Adoption of Electronic Medical Records. *Medscape Journal of Medicine,* Malaysian Multimedia Supercorridor at <http://www.mdc.com.my>

Maheu, M., Pulier. M., Wilhelm, F., McMenamin, J., and N. Brown-Connolly. (2005). *The Mental Health Professional and the New Technologies: A handbook for Practice Today.* New Jersey: Erlbaum.

Marks, I. M., Baer, L. Greist, J. H. et al. (1998). CIMH: Home self-assessment and self-treatment of obsessive compulsive disorder using a manual and a computer-conducted telephone interview I: Two UK-US Studies. *British Journal of Psychiatry,* 172, 406-12. <http://www.ex.ac.uk/cimh/btstep.htm>

McInnes, A. (n.d.) *The Agency of the Infozone: Exploring the Effects of a Community Network.*

Moore, G. E. (April 19, 1965). *Cramming more components onto integrated circuits.* Electronics Magazine, <http://www.firstmonday.dk/issues/issue2_2/mcinnes/index.html>

Murray, C. J., and Lopez, A. D. (eds.). (1996). *The Global Burden of Disease. A comprehensive assessment of mortality and disability from diseases, injuries and risk factors in 1990 and projected to 2020.* Harvard School of Public Health.

National Board for Certified Counselors. (1998). *NBCC Standards for the Ethical Practice of Webcounseling,* <http://www.nbcc.org/ethics/wcstandards.htm>

Neufeld, J. D., Yellowlees, P. M., Hilty, D., Cobb, H., and Bourgeois, J. A. (2007). The eMental Health Consultation Service: Providing enhanced primary-care mental health services through Telemedicine. *Psychosomatics,* 48, 35-141.

Nesbitt, T., Yellowlees, P., Hilty, D., and Hogarth, M. (Fall 2004). *Rural Health Care Technologies.* Institute of Medicine Rural Health Monograph.

Newman, M. G. (n.d.). *The Clinical Use of Palmtop Computers in the Treatment of Generalized Anxiety Disorder.*

Newman, M. G., Consoli, A., and Taylor, C. Barr. (1997). Computers in Assessment and Cognitive Behavioral Treatment of Clinical Disorders: Anxiety as a Case in Point. *Behavior Therapy,* 28, 211-235.

New Media Consortium. (Spring 2007). *Survey: Educators in Second Life.* <http://www.nmc.org/pdf/2007-sl-survey-summary.pdf.> Last accessed (January 3, 2008).

Newman, M.G., Kenardy, J., Herman, S., and Taylor, C. B. (February 1997). Comparison of palm-top computer –assisted brief cognitive behavioral treatment to cognitive behavioral treatment of panic disorder. *Journal Consultation Clinical Psychology,* 65(1), 178-83.

Oakley-Browne, M. A., and Toole, S. (1996). *Computerised self-care programs for depression and anxiety disorders.* Geneva, Switzerland: WHO.

Pellerin, C. (May 9, 2007). *U.S. Government Presence Grows in Second Life Online World.* The United States Mission to the European Union. <http://useu.usmission.gov.> Last accessed (October 4, 2007).

Perednia, D. (Feb 8, 1995). Telemedicine Technology and Clinical Applications. *The Journal of the American Medical Association,* 273(6).

Pickhardt, P. J., Choi, J. R., Hwang, I., Butler, J. A., Puckett, M. L., and Hildebrand, H. A., et al. (2003). Computed tomographic virtual colonoscopy to screen for colorectal neoplasia in asymptomatic adults. *N Engl J Med,* 349, 2191-2200.

Polauf, J. (1998). "Psychotherapy on the Internet – Theory and Technique." <http://www.nyreferrals.com/psychotherapy/>

Powell, T. (1998). "Online Counseling: A Profile and Descriptive Analysis." <http://netpsych.com/Powell.htm>

Rind, D., and Safran, C. (1994). *Real and Imagined Barriers to an Electronic Medical Record.* Reprinted from Seventeenth Annual Symposium on Computer Applications in Medical Care.

Rosen, E. (1998). Personal Telemedicine. *Telemedicine Today* (February), 10-13.

Rosen, E. (1997). Current Uses of Desktop Telemedicine. *Telemedicine Today* (March/April).

Rosen, J., Grigg, E., Lanier, J., McGrath, S., Lillibridge, S., Sargent, D., and Koop, C. E. (September/October 2003). The future of command and control for disaster response: Utilizing information and virtual reality technology, the Cybercare System can link resources throughout the country for distributed yet coordinated command and control. *IEEE Eng.,* 56-68.

Rosen, L. D., and Weil, M. M. (1997). Technostress: coping with *technology@ work@home@play*. New Jersey: John Wiley and Sons

Roy, M. J., Sticha, D. L., Kraus, P. L., and Olsen, D. E. (2006). Simulation and virtual reality in medical education and therapy: A protocol. *Cyberpsychol Behav*, 9, 245-7.

Sandom, C., and Harvey, R. S. (2004). *Human Factors for Engineers*. New York: Institution of Electrical Engineers.

Satava, R. M., and Jones, S. B. (Fall 1996). Virtual Reality and telemedicine: Exploring advanced concepts. Telemedicine Journal, 2(3), 195-200.

Slack, W. (1997). *Cybermedicine*. San Francisco: Jossey-Bass.

Spielberg, A. R. (Oct 21, 1998). On Call and Online – Sociohistorical, Legal, and Ethical Implications of E-mail for the Patient-Physician Relationship. *Journal of the American Medical Association*, 280(15).

Srinivasan, M., Yellowlees, P., Hwang, J., West, D., and Keenan, C. (Nov 2006). Assessment of Clinical Skills using Simulator Technologies. *Academic Psychiatry*, 30 (6), 505-515

Stofle, G. *Thoughts About Online Psychotherapy: Ethical and Practical Considerations* <http://members.aol.com/stofle/onlinepsych.htm>

Suler, J. (1996). The Psychology of Cyberspace at <http://www1.rider.edu> and at <http://www.behaviour.net>

Swartz, D. (1997). Healthcare moves to the Web. *Telemedicine Today* (December), 36-37.

Thompson, P. Medical Centers must find ways to reduce their environmental impact, and medical students can help. *The New Physician* (April 2008), 57(3). <http://www.amsa.org>. Accessed (April 30, 2008).

Van der Weyden, M. (December 7-21, 1998). Email: editors, doctors and patients. Medical Journal of Australia, 169(11-12), 571-2.

Viire, Erik. (July/August 1994). A Survey of Medical issues and Virtual Reality Technology. *Virtual Reality World*, 16-20.

Warner, D. J., (1997). The Globalization of Interventional Informatics Through Internet Mediated Distributed Medical Intelligence. Paper – Pulsar website.

Whitten, P., Collins, B., and Mair, F. (1998). Nurse and patient reactions to a developmental home telecare system. *Journal of Telemedicine and Telecare*, 4(3), 152-160.

Wootton, R., Yellowlees, P., and McLaren. P. (eds). (2003). *Telepsychiatry and e-Mental Health*. London: Royal Society of Medicine Press.

Wootton, R. et al. (1998). A joint US-UK study of home telenursing. *Journal of Telemedicine and Telecare*, 4 (Suppl.1), 83-85.

Wootton, R., and Darkins, A. (November-December 1997). Telemedicine and the doctor-patient relationship. *J R Coll Physicians Lond.*, 31(6), 598-9.

Wright, D. (1998). Telemedicine and Developing countries. *Journal of Telemedicine and Telecare,* 4(2), 1-88

Wootton, R., Dimmick, S., and Kvedar, J. (2006). *Home Telehealth: connecting care within the community.* London: RSM Press.

Wyatt, J., and Keen, J. (1998). The NHS's New Information Strategy. <http://www.bmj.com/cgi/content/full/317/7163/900>

Yale University School of Medicine Department of Surgery. *The NASA Commercial Space Center at Yale University Medical Informatics & Technology Applications* (MITA). <http://Yalesurgery.med.yale.edu/CSC/mita.htm>

Yatim, L. (1997). An Israeli telenursing call center: Home cardiac telemonitoring: Revisiting Israel's Shahal. *Telemedicine Today* (December), 26-33(4), 224-6.

Yellowlees, P. (1997). Successful development of telemedicine systems – seven core principles. *Journal of Telemedicine and Telecare,* 3, 215-222.

Yellowlees, P. (2005). Successfully Developing a Telemedicine System. *Journal of Telemedicine and Telecare,* 11, 331-335.

Yellowlees, P. M., and Brooks, P. M. (1999). Health online: the future isn't what it used to be. *Med J Aust,* 171, 522-5.

Yellowlees, P. M., and Cook, J. F. (2006). Education about hallucinations using an Internet virtual reality system: A qualitative survey. *Acad Psychiatry,* 30, 534-9.

Yellowlees, P., Hilty, D., and Odor, A. Cross-cultural store and forward telepsychiatry, <http://www.ucdmc.ucdavis.edu/psychiatry/research/technology.html>

Yellowlees, P., and Marks, S. (Nov 2006). Commentary: Pedagogy and Educational Technologies of the Future. *Academic Psychiatry,* 30(6), 439-441.

Yellowlees, P., and Harry, D. (Aug 2006). What standards should we develop for collection of data about telemedicine encounters to better facilitate research? *J Telemed and Telecare,* 12(Supp 2), 72-6.

Yellowlees, P., Hogarth, M., and Hilty, D. (Nov 2006). The Importance of Distributed Broadband Networks to Academic BioMedical Research and Education Program. *Academic Psychiatry,* 30(6), 451-455.

Yellowlees, P. M., and Marks, S. (2007). S Problematic Internet Use, or Internet Addiction? *Computers in Human Behavior,* 23, 1447-1453.

Yellowlees, P., and Marks, S. (2008) Can Virtual Reality be used to Conduct Mass

Prophylaxis Clinic Training? A Pilot Program. *Biosecurity and Bioterrorism.*

Yellowlees, P. (2008). Green Healthcare – why not? Web Video Editorial. *Medscape Journal of Medicine.*

Yellowlees, P. (2008). Green Healthcare – what is happening now? Web Video Editorial. *Medscape Journal of Medicine.*

Yellowlees, P. (2008). Green Healthcare – what does the future hold? Web Video Editorial. *Medscape Journal of Medicine.*

Young, K. (1998). Caught in the Net: how to recognize the signs of Internet addiction. New Jersey: John Wiley and Sons

Young, K. The Centre for On-Line Addiction, at <http://*www.netaddiction.com*>

Zajtchuk, R., and Satava, R. M. Medical Applications of Virtual Reality. Communications of the Association for Computing Machinery, 40 63-4

Printed in the United States
151328LV00020B/143/P

9 780595 527755